# HEALTH FINANCE *and* FINANCIAL MANAGEMENT

## Essentials for Advanced Practice Nurses and Interdisciplinary Care Teams

Mary A. Paterson, PhD, RN

*Ordinary Professor, School of Nursing*
*The Catholic University of America*
*Washington, DC*

Technical Editor
*Alexander V. Telyukov, PhD*

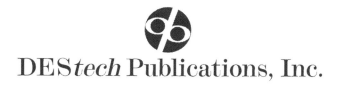

**DEStech Publications, Inc.**

# Healthcare Finance and Financial Management

DEStech Publications, Inc.
439 North Duke Street
Lancaster, Pennsylvania 17602 U.S.A.

Printed in the United States of America
10   9   8   7   6   5   4   3   2

Main entry under title:
    Healthcare Finance and Financial Management: Essentials for Advanced Practice Nurses
    and Interdisciplinary Care Teams

A DEStech Publications book
Bibliography: p.
Includes index p. 201

Library of Congress Catalog Card No. 2014931017
ISBN No. 978-1-60595-062-4

---

**HOW TO ORDER THIS BOOK**

BY PHONE: 877-500-4337 or 717-290-1660, 9AM–5PM Eastern Time

BY FAX: 717-509-6100

BY MAIL: Order Department
DEStech Publications, Inc.
439 North Duke Street
Lancaster, PA 17602, U.S.A.

BY CREDIT CARD: American Express, VISA, MasterCard, Discover

BY WWW SITE: http://www.destechpub.com

---

# Table of Contents

# Preface

**H**EALTHCARE in the United States is a complex blend of private, state, and federal systems with conflicting incentives that result in seemingly irrational financing policies. Over the more than twenty years that I have taught healthcare finance to clinical professionals, I have struggled to explain these systems in the short time allocated to this subject in a clinical program. The available healthcare finance textbooks are usually not intended for clinical students; they are either overly complex or too narrowly focused on the hospital enterprise or the entire healthcare financing system. This book provides an introduction to the healthcare financing system and a guide to the financial management of a healthcare practice. The book supports a semester-long class that prepares clinicians to participate knowledgeably in practice financial management and understand general concepts of the U.S. healthcare financing system.

The book is divided into two main sections. The first introduces the financing system, general models of healthcare financing with a focus on the concepts of risk and return, and health insurance models. The section concludes with a discussion of financial incentives and how they shape the costs of care. The second section focuses on financial management of the ambulatory care practice. This section provides a guide to cost finding, revenue analysis and management, and financial reporting. It concludes with two chapters focused on the planning, financial management, and evaluation of projects. These two chapters support not only capital investment analysis but also investment decisions on funded projects that the practice is considering. Taken together, the sections develop an understanding of the financing environment surrounding any clinical practice, the reasons for the state and federal financing policies with which a typical ambulatory care practice needs to comply, and the future challenges that are likely to develop given the new directions healthcare financing is taking with the Patient Protection and Affordable Care Act. Additionally, the book provides the practitioner with the basic financial tools necessary to survive as a business. The cases at the end of each section enable students to apply the material to practical problems in healthcare finance at the system and practice levels.

Healthcare finance is frequently taught in clinical programs by faculty who are not financial specialists. I provide simple, jargon-free explanations and examples to clarify financial theory and principles. I also provide an extensive instructor's manual with model syllabi, guides to all the cases, explanations of the problem sets, and PowerPoint slides intended to present the essential material in each chapter. Additionally, each chapter begins with clearly specified instructional objectives so that the material can be adapted to online instruction as well as classroom presentation. Students are provided with a review of essential concepts necessary to complete the chapter, along with study questions and problem sets that reinforce the material. The material is appropriate for a graduate class in healthcare finance, for clinical professionals such as nurse practitioners, physician's assistants, physical or occupational therapists, clinical psychologists, and social workers. It would also be applicable to graduate physicians interested in ambulatory care practice.

It has been both a challenge and a pleasure to compile this text with the clinical faculty and student in mind. I believe that well-informed clinical professionals are our best hope for a responsive and financially viable healthcare system. I wish all who use this book well as they begin the study of healthcare finance.

# Acknowledgments

THE material presented in this book is the result of a thirty-year dialogue with my teachers and students. I have found that the best education is a conversation between those who understand and those who seek to understand. This conversation is exciting, challenging, at times frustrating, and, above all, enlightening. This book could not have been written without my teachers, particularly Dr. Kyle Grazier, formerly at the University of California, Berkeley, and now at the University of Michigan, Ann Arbor. It could also not have been written without the many students who worked to understand, asked excellent questions, and insisted on clarity and simplicity. I am most grateful to them, but especially to the Doctor of Nursing Practice students at The Catholic University of America who pilot-tested much of this material when it was in draft form.

The educational dialogue between teacher and student is supported by our families. I thank my family and friends for their unfailing support of this work and the enrichment they bring to my life.

Finally I thank my colleagues at The Catholic University of America and at the American Association of Colleges of Nursing for their patience and forbearance as I struggled to complete this book, most especially to Dean Patricia McMullen who gave me the precious gift of time to focus on this project. I am grateful to all of you.

# Section 1

# CHAPTER 1

# Introduction to Healthcare Finance

## 1.1. Chapter Objectives

After completing this chapter you should be able to:

1. Define the terms *macro-finance* and *micro-finance*.
2. Discuss why healthcare providers need to know basic principles of financial economics.
3. Understand why government healthcare systems in the United States always have a political as well as administrative dimension.
4. Discuss the concept of states' rights and its implications for government healthcare systems.
5. Understand the evolving social compact in U.S. society in regards to healthcare financing.
6. Discuss the resource allocation issues inherent in the societal goal of health and healthcare.

## 1.2. What Do Healthcare Providers Need to Know about Finance and Financial Policy?

Economic theories are the basis for the concepts and principles that explain financial decisions. As students in healthcare fields, we may learn these principles as part of the required social science courses that we take before entry to professional study. Beginning healthcare students often find these concepts vaguely interesting but not very relevant for the work they intend to do. It is only after entry into practice that the impact of healthcare financing systems becomes apparent. For most of us, financial issues present barriers and constraints to what we consider the optimal delivery of care, and we decide that we need a better understanding of why the healthcare financing system seems to function the way it does.

This book is intended to help healthcare practitioners develop a better understanding of healthcare finance. It answers basic questions providers have concerning healthcare finance. The intention is not to develop a deep analytical expertise in accounting and finance; rather we provide an introduction to the main principles of healthcare financial policy and to some of the financial skills necessary to organize an effective and efficient professional practice. Most healthcare providers are also involved in making healthcare policy and allocation decisions—as voters as well as providers of care. So we begin with discussion of macro-finance. This area of finance is concerned with the way financial policy affects various sectors of the economy. Later sections of the book offer basic financial management knowledge that can help providers better organize their practice and make sound business decisions. This area of study is known as micro-finance.

The principles of financial economics help shape the way healthcare resources are managed in our society. For example, as providers of care, the amount and timing of the payment we receive for our services is determined by the financial realities of the healthcare sector. The distribution of healthcare to our patients is also determined by financial policy; whether services are paid or delivered pro bono, healthcare providers need to receive some payment for the work they do. The source, amount, and method of payment are all subject to many variations. Understanding financial economic and policy principles helps clarify not only the variations, but also the reasons for them.

### 1.3.  Characteristics of Financial Systems in Healthcare— The Social Compact

The effect of the financial system on the distribution of healthcare has been the topic of many research projects, policy briefs, books, and dissertations. The U.S. approach to healthcare financing is shaped by a few fundamental ideas that reflect the social compact between U.S. citizens and their government. One of the most important of these ideas is the relationship of the government to the people expressed clearly in this passage from the Declaration of Independence:

> We hold these truths to be self-evident, that all men are created equal, that they are endowed by their Creator with certain unalienable Rights, that among these are Life, Liberty and the pursuit of Happiness.—That to secure these rights, Governments are instituted among Men, deriving their just powers from the consent of the governed.

This compelling statement defines the way the government relates to the people. It derives from ideas discussed by social philosophers of the time, such as John Locke, Thomas Hobbs, and Jean-Jacques Rousseau. These individuals believed that people come together and agree to give up some of their individual liberty in exchange for benefits from a government that creates an orderly society for the good of all. However, if people judge that the government no longer serves the common good, individuals may act to change it. This relationship makes clear that the government serves the collective will of the people. If it does not, the people are free to change it.

The Declaration of Independence states that the fundamental power is with the people who agree to allow the government some role in supporting societal order. This arrangement implies that the people must agree with actions that the government takes on their behalf. Unlike governmental systems that concentrate power in a central government that may grant some rights to individuals, the U.S. system concentrates power with the individuals who grant rights to the government. This is an important allocation of power that has profound implications for any government healthcare system in the United States. In this country the people have the right to agree or disagree with any system of health insurance or healthcare that the government offers, and they also have the right to change it if they are not satisfied. Government healthcare systems in the United States are always subject to the will of the people and must have the approval of the majority of them in order to continue to exist. It is apparent, then, that government-managed healthcare will always have a political as well as an administrative aspect, and both are important if the system is to be sustainable.

A second important concept inherent in the U.S. system of government is the division between the rights and duties of state government and those of the federal government. The U.S. Constitution clearly establishes a federalist system that allocates only specific powers to the federal government. Powers not specifically given to the federal government remain with the states or with the people. The Tenth Amendment to the Constitution, often held to be redundant to reinforce ideas already inherent in the document's main body, makes this division of power unambiguous: "The powers not delegated to the United States by the Constitution, nor prohibited by it to the States, are reserved to the States respectively, or to the people."

The powers explicitly allocated to the federal government do not contain a reference to the establishment of healthcare or the right to healthcare; the involvement of the federal government in healthcare has been voluntary. For example, the establishment of federal programs to support care for active duty military and veterans, the Medicare program for the elderly, and the control of communicable disease were all established by Congressional action that contained no underlying mandate to provide health services for everyone. In fact, the federal government's right to regulate across state lines, including the right to tax and spend for the general welfare, stems from the commerce clause of the Constitution (Leonard, 2010). Constitutional scholars and the courts generally agree that health, welfare, and domestic safety are outside the boundaries of the commerce clause; therefore fall clearly within the powers reserved for the states. This is the reason that most government health programs in the United States have historically been the responsibility of the states, not the federal government.

These key concepts illustrate the critical relationship of the individual to the government in the United States and elucidate the social compact that exists in regard to healthcare. Individuals generally expect to provide healthcare for themselves, or in some cases to look to the state government for assistance. People historically do not expect the involvement of the federal government. Clearly, the advent of large federal programs such as Medicare and the significant federal share of Medicaid have changed this view. However, these relatively recent developments do not change the fundamental social agreements reflected in the documents that define the role of government in the United States. As shown in this brief discussion, historically there is a fundamental social understanding that the federal government has a limited and voluntary role in healthcare programs.

Given the social compact that exists in this society, healthcare financing can be expected to be primarily a private responsibility with some state involvement for vulnerable groups. The evolution of private health insurance, designed to assist individuals to bear the costs of healthcare services, reflects this societal expectation. Medicare and Medicaid, enacted in 1965, are relatively recent programs that reflect a new role for the federal government in financing the cost of care. The rapidly increasing number of individuals eligible for these programs has created an expanding health-financing role for government and accompanying financial requirements. The new mandates enacted in March 2010 with the passage of the Patient Protection and Affordable Care Act further increase the government's role in healthcare financing and promise to change further the expectations that U.S. citizens have for government involvement in the healthcare system.

The relatively recent emergence of this government role also illustrates the need for expanded fiscal policy and regulatory structures, many of which are not yet fully developed. Notably, some individuals do not agree with the expanded role of government and are challenging the constitutionality of these programs. The historic basis for these challenges and the importance of the changing social compact between individuals and the government in healthcare areas reflect the basic relationships we have discussed in this section.

## 1.4. Health or Healthcare—The Social Goal and the Financial Objective

As federal money is increasingly spent on healthcare, many policy makers have started to ask questions regarding the societal goals of these funds and press for accountability. Households have similar but less complex concerns regarding their private spending for healthcare. The household decisions can be made with careful consideration of the household's needs and resource allocations that match its members' preferences. These preferences are somewhat easier to determine in the smaller household unit. Spending tax monies for healthcare introduces a new level of complexity because societal welfare as a whole must be considered. Allocation strategies that focus on the greatest health gain that can be achieved for society may conflict with individual healthcare needs that also require the expenditure of public funds.

A classic dilemma in the allocation of public funds is the conflict between health and healthcare. More than thirty years ago, health economists posed this dilemma based on empirical analysis of the determinants of health in society (Fuchs, 1986, 274–279). If the goal for society is the overall health of its members, healthcare makes only a marginal contribution to health (Fuchs, 1986, 274; Newhouse and Friedlander, 1980). These early studies and many others have shown that strategies such as improving the educational level of society, improving the environment, and economic development in areas of poverty all make larger contributions to societal health than the delivery of healthcare. However, this does not remove the urgent need for individual healthcare when it is required. For most people improvement in education, environmental conditions, and economic development will not affect the conditions that require treatment now.

As government assumes the responsibility to pay for healthcare as well as create societal conditions that support health, financial allocation conflicts are certain to occur. The public health financing choices that ensue have no easy answer. For providers of healthcare, this dilemma has the following practical implications. Funds for healthcare are often found at the expense of reduced spending on education, environmental health, and social welfare. In this situation, healthcare providers still need to control healthcare spending but also deal with the adverse trends in public and personal health due to eroding social supports that create a healthy society. The classic example of the resulting conflict is the hospitalization of malnourished individuals to ensure that they have access to food. If the state raises money for acute care services by cutting back on social welfare programs such as nutrition support, the providers of care have to address the need for additional health services caused by severe malnourishment in their patients. Clearly from a cost-benefit perspective, it is far cheaper to provide food rather than finance increased hospitalization. However, at the point of serious malnutrition, it is too late to revisit more cost effective solutions. The provider must act to preserve life and does so at much greater expense. As this example illustrates, social allocation strategies that maximize health may do so at the expense of healthcare, while allocation strategies that maximize healthcare likely do so at the expense of long-term societal health. It remains a challenge for healthcare providers and public policy makers to find workable solutions to this dilemma and develop a clearer societal consensus on the goals for public financing in and around the health sector.

In the 2010 federal budget, healthcare consumed a larger share of the federal budget than disease prevention, social welfare, or education programs. This reflects the federal focus on large healthcare delivery programs such as Medicare, Medicaid, and the military healthcare systems. In fact, the only level of government that spends more on education than on health, education being a powerful determinant of long-term societal health, is the local government as can be understood from Figure 1.1. However, the local level represents the smallest share of the total of public monies expended on social programs, and it does not compensate for the lower spending on education seen at the state and federal level.

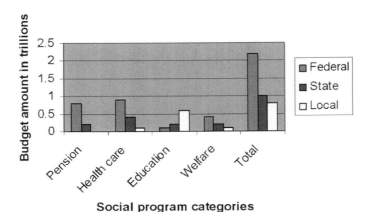

**Social program categories**

*FIGURE 1.1. Public spending estimates 2012. Source: Spending estimates compiled by C. Chantrill.*

Clearly, the dominant social spending objective at federal and state levels at the present time is healthcare, with less emphasis on programs that contribute directly to long-term population health such as education and social welfare. The long-term effects of this public allocation strategy pose risks for the overall health of society, which in turn will increase the demand for healthcare services.

## 1.5. Concept Checkout

Be sure you understand these concepts before you attempt the discussion questions:

- Macro-finance and micro-finance
- Financial economics
- Allocation of power to government and to people
- States' rights
- Health or healthcare as a societal objective

## 1.6. Discussion Questions

1. What is the main difference between macro-finance and micro-finance concepts? Conduct some independent research and find an example or an application of each concept.
2. Find a recent example of the debate between states and the federal government in regard to healthcare. This could be a court case involving states' rights or an administrative action between a state and the federal government.
3. You have learned that in the United States, power belongs to the people, who choose to allow government to act on their behalf. Find an example of another type of shared power between people and their government and contrast it with that of the United States, with a focus on government healthcare programs.
4. Give an example of and discuss the allocation dilemmas that occur as a result of the government's need to support either health or healthcare. For example, if the government chooses to support healthcare from a limited budget, does it reduce support of the population's overall health? Support your answer with evidence.
5. The Constitution states that the people have a right to change the government if they are not satisfied with it. This implies that people must be generally satisfied with systems instituted by the government on their behalf. How might this implication change your behavior as a provider of healthcare in a government-financed program?

## 1.7. References

Chantrill, C. Comparative spending at levels of government. (February 2012). Retrieved from www.usgovernmentspending.com/total_spending_2012USrn.

Budget of the U.S. Government, Fiscal Year 2010. Retrieved from www.gpo.gov/fdsys/pkg/BUDGET-2010-SUMMARY/pdf/BUDGET-2010-SUMMARY.pdf.

Fuchs, Victor. 1986. *The Health Economy.* Cambridge, Mass: Harvard University Press.

Leonard, Elizabeth Weeks. 2010. "State Constitutionalism and the Right to Health Care." *University of Pennsylvania Journal of Constitutional Law* 12: 1325–54.

Newhouse, Joseph P., and Friedlander, L. J. 1980. "The Relationship between Medical Resources and Measures of Health: Some Additional Evidence." *Journal of Human Resources* 15 (Spring): 200–218.

# CHAPTER 2

# Models of Healthcare Financing

## 2.1. Chapter Objectives

After completing this chapter you should be able to:

1. Define the key stakeholders in all health-financing models.
2. Discuss the role of the major stakeholders in healthcare financing.
3. Define the essential features of the major financing models: social insurance, private insurance, or out-of-pocket household payment.
4. Analyze the financial flows in each of the major financing models.
5. Assess the risks and benefits inherent in selected healthcare financing approaches.

## 2.2. The Household as a Central Stakeholder in Healthcare

In the first chapter we discussed the primary role of the household in the political structure of the United States. The influential position of the household is also central to understanding the evolution of health financing in this country. The household is the source of the funds that flow to all levels of government in the form of taxes and fees for public services, and these revenues enable the government to function. Figure 2.1 illustrates the importance of taxes as a source of government revenue. If government requires more money than households can provide, it will borrow by selling government bonds. Households in the United States can purchase these bonds and become government bondholders, as can other organizations and governments. Thus households not only provide government with revenue, they are also one of the primary sources of

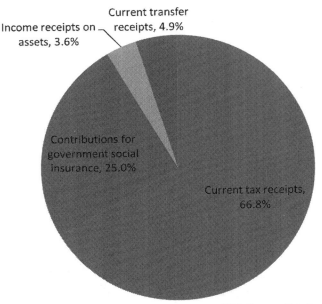

*FIGURE 2.1. Revenue sources for all levels of government, 2010. Source: U.S. Dept. of Commerce.*

funds when the government wishes to borrow money. Finally, the interest necessary to service this government debt is provided through taxation revenue. The household is an important financing and lending source for all levels of government. This is why households are critical stakeholders in health financing.

## 2.3. The Stakeholders in All Health-Financing Models

A review of the health-financing literature presents many possible financing arrangements used to pay for healthcare. Paying for healthcare is complex for many reasons. For example, we know that emergency healthcare services are lifesaving, and most societies agree that essential, lifesaving services should be available to all who need them, regardless of ability to pay. Emergency lifesaving care is considered differently than a broader-based right to essential nonemergency healthcare, which many countries, but not the United States, also include in their social compact. Urgent lifesaving services, such as care after an accident or major unplanned health event for example a heart attack or stroke, are usually provided in any society that has the capacity to provide such services. Payment for these essential services is collected after the emergency care has been provided. Where patients are expected to pay, the healthcare providers find themselves in a risky position because not everyone who receives emergency services can pay for them.

The information gap introduces another complexity. The average user of healthcare lacks the knowledge and training necessary to understand what services are required and cannot easily compare the cost and quality of the choices. This means that consumers need agents who can assist them to make informed choices. These agents can be primary care physicians, insurance company consumer representatives, specialist physicians, nurses, or other individuals with sufficient knowledge to assist the consumer in making healthcare choices. When consumers must use agents to make purchase decisions, there can be problems. Agents can serve interests other than the consumer and act in collusion with the provider group or the insurer, or they can simply fail to provide the consumer with a full menu of choices due to biases or deficits in their own knowledge base.

Issues such as the need to deliver emergency services and collect payment later or the need for agents to assist the consumer in making purchase choices have to be considered when health-financing systems are designed. These requirements often result in highly complex financing arrangements, for example, the need for a second opinion before a surgery or the requirement to obtain preauthorization before an emergency room visit is reimbursed. Regardless of these system complexities, healthcare objectives are clear: adequate access, acceptable quality, and affordable cost. It is generally agreed that healthcare systems can usually meet two of these three objectives, but meeting all three simultaneously has proved extremely difficult.

The stakeholders who must negotiate healthcare financing arrangements can be placed in one of four categories: government, private agents who act for the consumer, healthcare providers, and consumers, who are organized into households. All healthcare systems consider these stakeholder categories and design financing arrangements that involve all of them. Even systems that are fully privatized still have some government regulation for healthcare services, and systems that emphasize a single government payer have some private agents who act for the consumer, particularly consumers who choose to pay out-of-pocket for services either within the country or internationally. Table 2.1 provides a view of some of the actors in each of these stakeholder categories.

Table 2.1 is not an exhaustive list, but it provides insight into the mutiplicity of stakeholders in the U.S. healthcare system. The diverse cast of stakeholders is involved in health financing worldwide. The typology of health financing around the developed world is presented in Table 2.2 in the next section.

TABLE 2.1. *Stakeholders in the U.S. Healthcare System.*

| Governments | Healthcare Providers | Private Agents | Households |
|---|---|---|---|
| Federal government | Physicians and physician extenders such as physician assistants | Private insurance companies | Families |
| Military, including veterans care | Nurses including advanced practice nurses | Health Maintenance Organizations | Individuals in group-living situations with a caretaker. For example, adults/seniors/halfway houses. |
| U.S. Public Health Service Corps | Dentists | Consumer-focused special interest groups such AARP, Cancer Society, American Heart Association | Single individuals, including emancipated minors. |
| State government | Allied health personnel: laboratories, medical-device manufacturers, pharmacists, other diagnostic services | Employers | Individuals in cooperative residences such as communes, religious communities, mission-focused group living. |
| Local government | Residential and rehabilitation care facilities (nursing homes, protected-living providers, physical therapy providers) for profit and non-profit hospitals and hospital systems | Health-plan administrators/TPAs (used by self-insured employers) | |
| Regional government groups (As for example state alliances for information sharing, municipal and state alliances) | Rehabilitation facilities (skilled facilities, physical therapy, vocational rehabilitation) | Personal health consultants and other professionals contracted directly by the household | |
| | Provider-focused charitable organizations and foundations | Consumer-focused charitable organizations/donor groups | |

## 2.4.  The Essential Approaches to Healthcare Financing

The health care financing systems are defined by the mode of participation (mandatory or voluntary), benefit entitlement (contributory or non-contributory), method of raising funds (e.g., general taxes, earmarked contributions), scope of fund-pooling (from household to nation-wide level), finally, who has the authority to collect funds and use them to purchase healthcare. Table 2.2 explains the interplay of these criteria across the 34 developed economies, including the United States that are member states of OECD (Organization for Economic Cooperation and Development).

Notably, all the developed countries feature a blend of public and private approaches to healthcare financing. Any such country would self-identify with several if not most of the areas presented in Table 2.2.

There are two basic approaches to paying for healthcare: insurance and direct out-of-pocket payment. The most common choice for healthcare services is insurance because most individuals prefer to face a certain level payment rather than risk the financial uncertainty that accompanies direct payment when services are required. Health insurance may be provided exclusively through private markets, or the government may become involved either as a direct insurer or as a large purchaser of private insurance services. Socialized medicine, a situation in which the government assumes the roles of care provider and financier is a special case. In a completely socialized medicine, the government assumes all risk and assures the household of a set of healthcare services provided directly through government-owned hospitals and salaried providers. This approach is quite distinct from the social insurance case in which government provides insurance for some or all of the population but does not provide services directly.

To return to the U.S. healthcare system, financing health care services through private insurers is a system that was established in the United States during the early twentieth century. At the start, the cost of health services was low because little health technology existed. Hospitals were primarily places that provided care when home care was not available. For this reason, households saw little need for health insurance coverage. Rather, they preferred insurance for lost income, which represented the greatest cost to households in the early twentieth century (Thomasson, 2002). As the cost of healthcare increased due to advances in medical science, better training of providers, and technology development, the average household began to look for health insurance. The impact of the Depression on consumer resources coupled with the increasing cost of healthcare was a strong influence on the development of private health insurance plans sold directly to households. A major

TABLE 2.2. The Global Typology of Health Care Financing.

| System Type | Participation | Entitlement | Fund-raising | Fund-pooling | Financing Agents — Revenue Collection | Financing Agents — Healthcare Purchasing |
|---|---|---|---|---|---|---|
| National Health Service | Automatic for all citizens or target population (e.g., the poor), as defined by applicable law | Non-contributory, typically universal or based on eligibility criteria by target population | Mandatory funding, typically from general budget revenue (primarily taxes) | National, sub-national, by entitlement program | Government agencies | Government entities, NGOs, private entities |
| Social health insurance (SHI) | Mandatory for all citizens or target population groups | Contributory: based on payment by, or on behalf of the insured | Mandatory; risk-unrelated contributions. Governments usually pay for non-contributing populations | National, sub-national, by program; government may subsidize poor regions and population groups | Government agency, National Health Insurance Agency, Social health insurance funds, Private insurance companies | |
| Mandatory private insurance | Mandatory: for all citizens or target population groups | Contributory: an insurance policy from a designated or freely chosen insurance company is required | Insurance premiums, usually related to risk but not to income | By health insurance carrier and/or plan | Government entities, Social health insurance funds, private insurance companies | Private insurance companies, public organizations |
| Voluntary insurance | Voluntary | | | | | |
| Out-of-pocket expenditure | Voluntary (HSAs), or mandatory (deductibles, copay in SHI) | Contributory: service is provided to paying customers | From household disposable income and savings | By household | Insurance organizations, Providers of health care | |

Adapted from: OECD/WHO/Eurostat, 2011: A System of Health Accounts, 2011 Edition, Chapter 7: Classification of Health Care Financing Schemes: 163, 184 impetus to the development of employer-sponsored health insurance came as a result of wage and price controls during World War II. Fierce competition for available labor coupled with wage controls made non-cash employee benefits one of the few incentives employers could offer to attract workers. As a result, employer-sponsored health insurance as an employment benefit gained in popularity and became an expectation for most unionized and salaried employees in the United States. Today, the high cost of advanced healthcare technology makes some form of insurance coverage necessary for most citizens. Those who cannot afford to purchase insurance depend on state-provided benefits for the poor, or cross-subsidization from insured users of hospital services who pay the overhead costs of essential care delivered to those who cannot pay.

A major change in U.S. health financing occurred in 1965 with the advent of Medicare, a federal government program that insures the elderly, and Medicaid, which insures the poor. Medicare provides insurance for hospital care to individuals over sixty-five who are entitled to Social Security (Medicare Part A), and subsidized insurance for ambulatory care so that the elderly can access physicians (Medicare Part B). The newest addition to the Medicare plan is Part D, which covers a significant part of the cost of prescription drugs for the elderly. Medicaid is a shared program for the poor; the federal government assumes about half the cost of services and individual states assume the other half. Medicaid also is the major financing program for long-term care delivered to the low-income elderly.

The entry of the federal government into these major health insurance programs was an important milestone. Rather than a purely private system of health financing, the U.S. system became a blended one, with government assuming about half the cost of care through Medicare, Medicaid, federal worker insurance programs, and the military health service, which is an example of government-delivered and financed healthcare.

Out-of-pocket payment to providers occurs in all healthcare systems. In a social insurance system, government rules may allow individuals to opt-out of the government health sector and instead purchase services from private providers, as is the case in Canada. In most systems, households also incur out-of-pocket costs through copayments and deductibles, which are not part of the insurance payment. Out-of-pocket payments have two general functions in health-financing systems: (1) proven control of moral hazard, which occurs when households do not face the full cost of services and, as a result, over-utilize services that they perceive as low-cost and (2) a theoretical increase of sensitivity to both the quantity and quality of services delivered. (Rand Health,

2006). Findings from the Rand Health Insurance experiment unequivocally support the effect of cost sharing on service utilization; however, the effect of cost sharing on sensitivity to the quality of services is not supported. In theory, consumers who pay for care should exert direct influence on the quality of the care they receive. But the information gap between consumers, who lack training to accurately judge quality, and the provider may be too great for this effect to occur.

Many proponents of free-market solutions to the health-financing question have advocated for more direct payment for healthcare. The development of health savings accounts (HSAs), which allows individuals to shelter a portion of their income from tax and save it for healthcare expenses, is a current example of such an approach. The combination of the HSA and a catastrophic health insurance policy with a high-deductible level is envisioned as the solution to both over-utilization and high cost. The tax implications of this solution also make the public sector a stakeholder in the HSA because tax policy is a major factor in the HSA funding formula. The HSA approach uses market forces to sensitize the consumer to the true cost of care because the consumer pays out-of-pocket for most routine expenses. The evidence on the consumer's use of information to make wise healthcare purchase decisions is not definitive as yet, and the agency problem has not been solved. However, many proponents of HSAs believe that consumers will demand better information when they need it to make informed healthcare purchases.

## 2.5. The Financial Flows in Healthcare Systems

Our previous discussion has shown that the household provides the majority of funds for financing healthcare services. The transfer of these funds from the household to the providers of care can take many pathways. In the United States, the major conduits for health financing are private health insurers, the federal government, and state governments. As previously discussed, the household can pay for private health insurance that will, in turn, pay providers when care is required. Private health insurance operates on a risk-based financial model that uses actuarial tables to estimate risk and set health insurance premiums accordingly. These models will be studied later in this book. Governments either purchase health insurance from the private sector or becomes the insurer and uses public funds to finance health services for the population. If government serves as the guarantor of care, it may choose a risk-based financial model similar to private insurance. The government may also choose a budget model in which an annual amount is budgeted for healthcare, and when that amount is gone, no further funds are available. In this case, provider payment is delayed until the new government budget money is available. To avoid such a budget shortfall the government depends on the accuracy of forecasting models projections. Political pressures, the influence of special-interest groups, and intersectoral competition for government resources all exert pressure on budget-financed healthcare systems and may cause difficulties for providers depending on government payments. In all financing systems, control of provider cost is a major issue, together with assurance of adequate access and quality.

## 2.6. Concept Checkout

Be sure you understand the following concepts before you begin the discussion questions:

- Household role in U.S. health finance
- Major stakeholders in health finance
- Social insurance
- Socialized medicine
- Blended healthcare financing schemes
- Private out-of-pocket healthcare finance
- Flow of funds in health financing

## 2.7. Discussion Questions

1. Explain and give examples of the role of the household in U.S. healthcare financing.
2. You have been asked to survey the main stakeholders in a small state to ascertain their opinions about healthcare costs. List five stakeholder groups you will include and provide a rationale for including them.
3. Explain the concept of social insurance and give an example of a social health insurance system either in the United States or in another country. Include a general description of the funds flow in the system you select.
4. Analyze the health savings account approach to financing healthcare. Include in your analysis the following: definition of the HSA, tax treatment of HSA accounts, incentives to establish an HSA, and at least three strengths and weaknesses of the HSA approach.
5. Evaluate one healthcare financing system in the United States. It can be a state-level system, a federal system, a private system, or a blended system. Discuss at least three financial strengths and three financial weaknesses of the system.

## 2.8. References

OECF/WHO/Eurostat, 2011: A System of Health Accounts, 2011 Edition. OECD Publishing. Retrieved from http://www.keepeek.com/Digital-Asset-Management/ oecd/social-issues-migration-health/a-system-of-health-accounts/classification-of-health-care-financing-schemes-icha-hf_9789264116016-9-en#page3

Rand Corporation. 2006. "The Health Insurance Experiment." Retrieved from www. rand.org/content/dam/rand/pubs/research_briefs/2006/RAND_RB9174.pdf.

Thomasson, M. A. 2002. "From Sickness to Health: The Twentieth-Century Development of U.S. Health Insurance." *Explorations in Economic History* 39: 233–53.

U.S. Department of Commerce, Bureau of Economic Analysis. "Government Current Receipts and Expenditures." *National Income and Products Accounts Tables (2009–2011)*. www.bea.gov/national/nipaweb/TableView.asp?SelectedTable=86&Freq=Qt r&FirstYear=2009&LastYear=2011.

# The Island Nation of Tekram

*Before you begin this case be sure you have completed Chapters 1 and 2 in the text.*

Tekram is an island nation in the South Pacific. The climate is tropical and the nation is self-governing after a period of colonial rule by the British. The population of the island is 500,000, including permanent residents, 300,000 of whom are year-round residents. The remaining inhabitants claim Tekram citizenship but are seasonal residents only. There is one urban center with a population of 150,000. The rest of the population lives in small villages. The people support themselves with fishing and small-scale agriculture. They do not manufacture anything, so Tekram is dependent on trade and tourism for most of the necessities of life. The main trade products are tropical fruit and fish, and the main revenue source for the government is tourism and related industries such as hotels and restaurants. The island has one international airport and a deep-sea harbor that can accommodate ocean-going cruise ships and freighters. The island's energy needs are met by imported oil and a small domestic solar-power generating industry. Potable water is in short supply on the island and during periods of drought it must be imported in tankers.

The average family size on Tekram is six. The majority (70 percent) of households on the island are Christian, the rest either claim no religious affiliation or are Hindus, part of a small population of East Indians that migrated to Tekram during the British rule. The government is a parliamentary democracy patterned after the British system. The president is appointed every four years by the majority party. Tekram is divided into twenty parliamentary districts. Freeplace, the capital and

21

only city, has four of these districts. The average size of a district nationwide is 25,000 individuals or about 4,100 households. All citizens of Tekram may vote; those who are not full-time residents may vote by absentee ballots. The average participation rate in parliamentary elections is 48 percent. Elections must be held every four years but may be more often if the majority party declares an election or suffers a vote of no confidence in the parliament. There is a written constitution, a system of courts, and a small civil service with 5,000 employees. Parliament meets for eight months of each year. It is composed of a parliamentary council with committees for the government's major activities. Each committee is headed by a minister appointed by the majority party. Health has a separate committee, and there is a minister of health.

Health is a major issue on Tekram. When the nation was founded 30 years ago, the government owned all the health facilities, which had been built by the British. They provided free care to all of Tekram's citizens at these government clinics and hospitals. In Freeplace, Tekram founded a university with a medical and nursing school, but most graduates do not stay on the island, and there is a persistent shortage of nurses and physicians. This shortage, together with the increasing costs of technology and maintenance of the aging health infrastructure, has increased healthcare costs to a level that is unaffordable for the government. During the last parliamentary session, healthcare was moved to a social insurance system. The government is relinquishing management of all healthcare facilities to interested private individuals and organizations. The country's first private hospital was opened this year by the Church of England as a nonprofit facility providing care to all. Missionary doctors and nurses makeup the majority of the staff, but Tekram health providers also work at the hospital. While the hospital is committed to giving care to all who need it, the management team knows that all care cannot be provided below cost. The government of Tekram has invited a U.S.-based managed care organization to provide an HMO-model insurance plan to Tekram. Through contributions to the social insurance scheme, the government will provide safety-net coverage for the 15 percent of its citizens who fall below the poverty line. The rest of the population must purchase the insurance, either directly or through their employers. Health insurance coverage is mandatory. There is no requirement for employers to provide health insurance, so the majority of coverage is purchased by households or by the government for its employees and for the poor.

Since the citizens of Tekram are used to having the government provide health services at a low cost, they are becoming increasingly upset about the new scheme. They feel the cost of health insurance is too high and the coverage is not complete. For example, preventive care such as immunizations, routine physicals, and well-baby visits must be paid out-of-pocket. Elective procedures in the hospital and all diagnostic services carry a 20 percent co-payment, and there is a deductible of $200 per disease episode that must be paid regardless of the type of care that is provided. There is no long-term care available, nor is there any occupational health. Mental healthcare is provided if there is an acute mental illness for the 20 percent co-payment. Otherwise mental healthcare, counseling for substance abuse, and all other counseling is paid out-of-pocket. In general, the system provides and pays for essential acute hospital care, but it does not pay for preventive or rehabilitative care. It does not pay for long-term care for the elderly although there is a government old-age pension for former government employees and the poor.

Major health problems in Tekram include cardiovascular disease, stroke, diabetes, arthritis, tuberculosis, and motor-vehicle accidents. The HIV/AIDS rate is low, but the rate of tuberculosis is high in this population. The incidence rate has increased to 60 cases in the population, three of which are drug-resistant. The government has a public health office, and it is very concerned with decreasing the rate of infection for TB, avoiding the further development of drug-resistant TB, and increasing compliance with the antibiotic therapy for TB cases. The office is aware of the impact on tourism if TB gets any further out of control. It has instituted the directly observed therapy (DOTS) approach to the TB epidemic. Starting the DOTS program required an increase of one physician, one nurse, and one community health worker to the civil service in the health ministry. This increase has resulted in a parliamentary debate on government health expenditures because the new social insurance program, which provides acute care for the poor, already takes the entire dedicated health budget. The persistent budget overruns for the ministry of health are going to require either tax increases or cutting money from the ministries of education, social welfare, or the environment. The Tekram population has made it clear that a tax increase will result in considerable pressure on the parliament to change the government.

You are a consultant, hired by the Tekram ministry of health to provide guidance in this situation. You have been asked to formulate a strategy to address the current crisis in health spending. The ministry is most concerned with the lack of consensus in the Tekrami population on the health goals for the country. It has asked you to formulate a consensus-building strategy to increase agreement on the goals for the country's health system.

As you review the situation, you realize that the current literacy rate of only 40 percent has already impacted the capacity of citizens to understand the current health dilemma. In your opinion, funding for education cannot be further reduced. Reducing the budget for environmental services will impact the ability of the government to supply clean potable water to the population in times of drought. This, in turn, inevitably results in an increase in maternal and infant mortality due to water-borne parasites in the native water available. The TB epidemic must be controlled because of the economic dependence on tourism. Eighty percent of the social service budget is currently spent providing safety-net social insurance coverage for the poor, and there appears to be no support for decreasing that level of payment.

Your case analysis should answer the following questions:

1. What do you recommend as the basis for the new health strategy in Tekram. Discuss the reasons for your recommendation and the policy evidence from the literature that supports these recommendations.
2. State at least one goal and two objectives that are critical to your strategy. Your goal should be SMART (specific, measurable, attainable, realistic, and timely).
3. Make at least one recommendation on how to build support for your strategy.
4. Discuss at least three methods that the ministry should use to implement your support-building recommendation.
5. Suggest one alternative to the present social insurance scheme, and provide a rationale for the feasibility of this alternative.

You may make reasonable assumptions to support your case discussion; however, these assumptions should be consistent with your understanding of a poorly educated lower middle-class population that is dependent on service industries, subsistence agriculture, and fishing for a livelihood. For example, it would be unreasonable to assume that the population of Tekram could double their GDP in one year by advancing high-technology innovation. However, you might make an assumption that the government could encourage investment in some non-tourist industries if appropriate training infrastructure was developed for some of the population.

# Section 2

# CHAPTER 3

# Health Insurance in Public and Private Markets

## 3.1. Chapter Objectives

After completing this chapter you should be able to:

1. Explain the concept of risk in relation to health insurance.
2. Describe the basic actuarial formula and explain its use.
3. Define experience and community rating.
4. Describe the budget approach to health insurance.
5. Discuss the two major types of risk control strategies in health insurance.

## 3.2. The Nature of Risk

In the financial world, risk is equivalent to uncertainty. For example, a loan with a certain payback is considered much less risky than a loan for which payback is very uncertain. A lender's reward for higher risk is higher interest. Interest is the amount of money due to the lender for the use of its money, and interest is higher when loan payback is highly uncertain. This higher interest, due to uncertain payback, is often called the risk premium. In general, the less certain a financial event is, the riskier it is for investors. For example, a company entering a market for the first time lacks experience. If the company wishes to borrow money (issue bonds), it will pay a higher interest because investors lack information on how the company will perform and if it will repay the bond principal. Investors expect this risk premium because recovery of the principal is not certain and the higher interest payments they receive now compensate them for their future potential loss. On the opposite extreme, established companies with market experience usually pay a lower interest rate when they issue bonds. This is because investors have more information about the company's performance in the market, and they are far more certain that they will recover their principal.

In the health insurance market, the risk that accompanies uncertainty is also costly. In health insurance contracts, there are two principal stakeholders: the insurer and the insured.[1] Both stakeholders try to decrease the uncertainty involved in health insurance so that they can avoid unplanned expenses. Insurers want to be certain that they will set the premiums high enough to pay all claims, meet the cost of operating the insurance company, and make a fair profit. The members of a household purchase health insurance in order to be able to predict the payments they have to make for healthcare services and to avoid unexpected and very large payments.

Health insurance is usually an attractive product for a household. Even for healthy individuals, direct out-of-pocket payments for healthcare are far less predictable than a monthly premium for health insurance. If people could be certain of the timing and level of their healthcare expenses, they would purchase health insurance only when they expect costs higher than the premium. Needless to say, such a rational choice on the part of the insured would make the insurers' financial risk untenable; the insurer would never collect sufficient funds to pay all certain claims that households would make.

In reality there is no way to be certain of healthcare expenses. But both stakeholders want the most accurate estimate possible of the likely outlay of funds for healthcare so that they can make informed financial decisions. The more uncertain they are, the higher the risk premium in the health-insurance market and the more willing the household is to pay it if its members value a certain payout over the chance that they will be unexpectedly hit with a large healthcare bill. Some households value this certainty more than others do. In general, younger households with less disposable income prefer to take a chance, since they are generally healthy. Older households with more income and higher exposure to disease risks prefer to pay the risk premium in exchange for greater certainty about healthcare expenses. Health insurers always value health information because they can set premium rates more accurately. Households may not always wish health insurers to have this information, particularly if it will increase the health insurance premium.

---

[1]Employers and providers are also health insurance stakeholders and their role will be discussed later in the chapter.

## 3.3.  Estimating Risk in Health Insurance

Actuarial rating is the process of estimating the premiums that an individual or group must pay for health-insurance coverage. There are two general methods used to set the premiums: experience rating and community rating. In experience rating, the past utilization experience of the group is considered in setting the premium. Experience rating depends on accurate cost information and good assessments of the probability of health utilization, usually based on prior usage of services together with demographic information and current health history of the individuals applying for coverage. In experience rating, the premiums charged by health insurers are estimated using a set of actuarial formulas that focus on expected healthcare costs (risks) for the defined group. The basic considerations in experience rating are:

1. The projected amount of financial loss the group may have
2. The probability that the loss will actually happen
3. The administrative fee required to administer the insurance scheme

The basic formula to compute the premium in experience rating is:

If the *amount of loss* = $a$; the *probability of loss* = $b$;
the *fair administrative fee* = $c$;

Then the *premium for a defined group* = $(a \times b) + c$

Application of this basic actuarial formula illustrates some important concepts about risk in experience-rated health insurance.

The first concept illustrated by the basic formula is: it does not make financial sense to insure a certain event. As an example, let us assume that an individual knows that he or she will certainly have a healthcare event that will cost $600. Therefore the probability of that event occurring is 100 percent or 1.00. Use of the basic actuarial formula shows that the cost of purchasing insurance will be higher than simply saving $600 and paying when the time comes. Since the amount of loss equals $600 times 1.00 plus a fee for administration of the insurance, the fair insurance premium is greater than the cost of the event itself. There are some events that households try to insure for less than the full cost of the service, such as maternity care, planned elective surgeries, and preventive services. Health insurers respond with a variety of analytical and program design options, such as qualifying periods and exemptions for previously identified conditions, to avoid insuring certain events at less than full cost.

Other planned events decrease the cost of future covered services, for example effective preventive care can decrease future acute care costs. In these cases, insurers agree to cover the cost of the certain event at a discount in order to save on future costs. However, the insurer needs to retain the enrollee long enough to recoup the investment in the preventive service. This is one reason insurers are less willing to cover preventive services when groups can disenroll after short coverage contracts.

The second principle is: the larger and more similar the group, the more accurate the premium estimate will be. The fact that estimates become more stable with larger populations is an important factor in optimizing allocations in uncertain conditions (Artstein and Hart, 1981, 485). Another consideration is that large groups that share similar characteristics tend to exhibit more predictable health utilization patterns given the similarity of their health risks.

Health insurers incorporate these principles into health insurance policy design. For example, they know that individuals within a group may try to purchase insurance to cover certain events in the hope that the insurers will not accurately identify the event as certain and will set the premium lower. In our example, if the probability of $600-event was estimated at 0.9 instead of 1.00, the premium would be 540 plus the administrative fee. This would likely be a saving for the beneficiary and a loss for the insurer. This is one reason that policies are designed with qualifying periods and insurers exclude pre-existing conditions and services such as cosmetic surgery that are entirely at the consumer's discretion and do nothing to reduce the probability of future healthcare costs. Notice, however, that healthcare prevention like annual physical examinations, well-baby care, health screenings, or other preventive measures are covered by many insurers because they do impact the future level of disease-related healthcare costs. This stands to reason because, while the events are controlled by the consumer and may be certain to occur, they lower the probability of loss for more expensive illnesses that are usually covered in a standard health insurance policy. The insurer will be more willing to cover preventative services in a multiyear coverage contract because the likelihood of retaining the beneficiary long enough to benefit from covered preventive services increases with the contract duration. Medicare, a program that by law provides lifetime coverage to eligible retirees, has strong reasons to motivate their beneficiaries to use preventive services.

Insurers who use experience rating to establish premium rates will accept high-risk individuals if they can charge the actuarially fair premium for coverage because the premium would reflect the higher cost and probability of use. Thus it would not represent an automatic loss for the insurer. The disadvantage of the experience-rating method is that health insurance may become unaffordable for chronically ill individuals, who are likely to incur high healthcare costs.

In community rating, a system used by most Blue Cross plans, all members of a group are charged the same amount regardless of their healthcare utilization patterns. The premium is based on a budget-planning principle that estimates the community's future healthcare costs based on its historic expenses. The insurer then divides these costs by the size of the community, and each member pays a fair share of the projected healthcare cost regardless of individual utilization history. It has been noted that community rating in its pure form has never been used; from the beginning the Blue Cross plans divided the communities it covered into premium classes and tiers such as single, married, and married with children (Follman, 1962,406). These tiers paid different premiums depending on their historic utilization patterns and projected future costs. Blue Cross plans and federally qualified HMO plans use tiered premium rate structures that consider the utilization experience of each tier.

Community rating involves a social welfare approach to health insurance. Those who are chronically ill generally benefit from the community rate while those individuals who are healthy pay more than an actuarially fair premium based on their individual utilization experience. Further, if community rating is to work, the community must value healthcare for all so that low-cost individuals who pay higher premiums than their experience merits are willing to remain in the plan to subsidize the higher cost individuals. If lower cost individuals do not remain in the plan, a phenomenon known as adverse selection occurs. If only the most costly, sickest individuals are left in a community-rated plan, they have to pay more because there are fewer participating community members to share the costs of the insurance. Eventually only those who directly benefit from insurance are left in the plan, and their premiums reflect their utilization experience because no subsidization from the healthy to the sick is left.

That is why it is said that, in the end, all plans are experience-rated unless health insurance is mandatory and healthy individuals must remain in the insurance pool.

## 3.4.  Managing Costs as a Risk-Control Strategy

Health insurers have learned that the competitive health-insurance market will not accept unlimited escalation of premiums. Regardless of the approach to determining them, premiums are defined largely by the underlying cost of delivering covered healthcare services. The Department of Health and Human Services' Centers for Medicare and Medicaid Services (CMS) publishes healthcare expenditure projections based on major cost categories.

As an example, Figure 3.1 illustrates the expenditures for fiscal year 2012.

Hospital care and physician and clinical services are major cost-control targets because together they represent 62 percent of the annual expenditures. Health insurer's strategies to control these costs can be grouped into two general categories: supply-side control, such as management of care provided, and the cost of that management; and demand-side control, such as benefit and accessibility management. Management of the care provided includes strategies such as preferred-provider panels, stipulation of required provider qualifications, and direct utilization and case management designed to directly impact how care is provided to the beneficiary. Cost management generally focuses on rate schedules, negotiated discounts for services, and stipulation of certain technologies or classes of pharmaceuticals, such as generic drugs. Benefit management is the area that defines services that are covered and excluded. Expensive or experimental services with unproven outcomes are generally excluded to manage costs by constraining demand for these services. Accessibility management is sometimes known as queuing. By lengthening wait times for expensive elective procedures such as hip replacement or major organ transplants, costs are decreased. Both benefit management and queuing constrain the demand for care.

The insurance company is also expected to control their own admin-

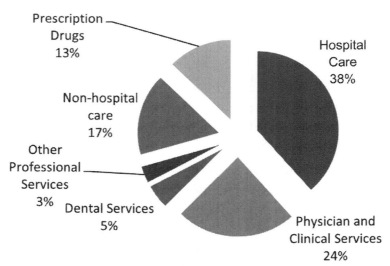

*FIGURE 3.1.* *Health expenditure categories, 2012. Source: Centers for Medicare and Medicaid Services*

istrative costs. The amount of administrative cost inherent in the U.S. healthcare system has been a topic of much discussion in the health policy community, particularly when U.S. administrative costs are compared to countries with national healthcare systems such as Canada or the United Kingdom. It is hard to dispute the fact that reported administrative costs in national health insurance programs are significantly lower than those under the blended public-private system in the United States. A careful comparison of the federal costs of administering Medicare and private insurance in the U.S. in 2006 found Medicare administrative costs to be slightly lower (Litow, 2006, 2). The report further describes the care that must be taken to compare government and private administrative cost categories as well as the methods necessary to compare such costs across the beneficiary or claims base.

Regardless of the public or private nature of the plan, administration of health-insurance systems is a relatively costly activity, and these costs must be taken into account when discussing premiums. The fact that in public plans more than one government agency pays the administrative costs obscures but does not remove this cost consideration. It is also important to understand that cost and compliance management require administrative expenditures. The more market pressure the health insurer experiences and the more highly regulated the industry becomes, the higher the administrative costs will be. All of these facts notwithstanding, both consumers and regulators expect that health insurers will keep administrative costs under control and behave efficiently. In this case, careful consideration needs to be given to the amount of cost and regulatory oversight for which beneficiaries are willing to pay.

### 3.5.  The Budget Approach to Health Insurance

Global budgets that limit the expenditure on healthcare services are a tool that can be used in either public or private systems. In some developing countries the entire public healthcare delivery system is managed with a global budget allocated from the government treasury to the ministry of health. The ministry, in turn, manages the salaries of the health workforce and purchases the supplies and physical resources necessary to delivery services in clinics and hospitals. The system is entirely managed from the supply side, and if demand exceeds the budgeted supply, care is either not available or is paid with under-the-table (informal) payments from consumers. In globally budgeted systems, these informal payments can also expedite care, pay for higher quality care, or pay for a particular provider. This is the system that was in place in the former Soviet Union, where it is estimated that approximately one-third of provider income came from informal payments (Telyukov, 2010).

Global budgets are also used in private insurance systems that either directly own healthcare facilities, for example HMOs such as Kaiser Permanente, or that enter into capitated rate arrangements with preferred providers. In capitated rate arrangements, providers agree to give all necessary care to an assigned panel in exchange for a flat payment per panel enrollee. These arrangements shift the risk to the provider in exchange for a capped budget. The idealistic principle underlying a global budget is that providers will seek to manage the risk of exceeding the budget by preventing serious illness in the assigned panel. In reality, there are considerable incentives for providers simply to deny necessary care in order to stay within the global budget. Where healthcare costs are controlled by means of global budgets, demand for care cannot be fully met. In this type of system families should consider healthy lifestyles as a priority goal.

The major social determinants of health such as education, environment, and social welfare become important to the family when healthcare is controlled by a global budget.

### 3.6.  Risk Control Strategies in Health Insurance

The options available to the health insurer to control risk derive directly from the sources of risk described in the basic actuarial formula presented earlier. To manage risk, the health insurer needs to consider managing the probability and amount of loss. These categories are not mutually exclusive. For example, a screening test that detects cancer in an earlier stage may decrease the probability of loss because major surgery may not be required to remove the lesion. The same screening test certainly decreases the amount of loss because excision of a small lesion is far less expensive than a major surgical resection and adjuvant chemotherapy that is normally recommended in the case of a larger tumor.

In general, the insurer focuses on preventive strategies that are likely to pay back the expense of the strategy. It is easy to appreciate the dilemma that a private insurer faces when considering preventive programs that are relatively expensive and unlikely to pay back in a short time. Because health insurance is tied to employment for the majority of the U.S. population under 65 years of age, tenure in a given job provides some guidance to health insurers of the time horizon required to benefit from prevention programs. A recent review of job tenure in the United States confirms two important trends: a decline in long-term job tenure and an increase in short-term employment (Farber, 2010). These trends increase the dilemma for the insurer interested in payback on prevention programs. Even if the insurer is successful in retaining the employer as a client, it is not likely that the employee will be there long enough to pay back the expense of high-cost prevention programs. The role of regulatory actions to level the playing field for all insurers is important in this discussion. If all insurers are required to cover proven preventive procedures, then the odds of receiving a new enrollee who is current with preventive care increases, and the insurer's investment in preventive services is not unique.

Management of the amount of loss is a more amenable challenge, and insurers have focused on these strategies for many years. Negotiated discounts from providers, the use of preferred diagnostic service providers, and the use of generic drugs whenever possible are all examples of strategies used to control the amount of loss. Large claims management, used more often with claims that exceed a million dollars, is also a way of decreasing the probability of large losses.

The promise of electronic medical records is that both the amount and probability of loss decrease as providers understand the totality of an individual's medical history and manage both preventive and episodic care with more precision. As billing, auditing, and claims management become integrated with clinical documentation, electronic medical records also promise to decrease administrative costs. It is no surprise that health insurers and regulators are focused on early adoption of this promising technology despite its cost. Providers, on the other hand, do not receive the savings from the use of the electronic medical records, but they incur the cost. This is one reason providers are less convinced that electronic documentation is a good investment.

In summary, the basic actuarial equation that relates premiums to the amount and probability of loss is the foundation for understanding risk and risk management in the health-insurance industry. Private and public health insurers must manage the sources of risk as well as contain the administrative cost of providing coverage in order to assure an efficient health-insurance service.

## 3.7.  Concept Checkout

Be sure you understand the following concepts before you begin the discussion questions:

- Health-insurance risk
- Basic actuarial equation
- Experience rating
- Community rating
- Cost management in health insurance
- Global budgets
- Risk-control strategies

## 3.8. Discussion Questions

1. The promise of genomic medicine is that the uncertainty surrounding individual health risks will be greatly reduced. By understanding each individual's genetic map, the risks of certain chronic diseases can be estimated for the individual with great precision. Discuss at least two major impacts genomics may have on health-insurance risk from the perspective of the insurer. *Assume that the insurer is not allowed access to an individual's specific genetic map.*

2. A state legislator has suggested that the community-rating method be required for all insurers writing health-insurance policies in her state. She belongs to a political party that does not accept the principle of mandatory health insurance. Do you think the community-rating requirement will make a difference to health-insurance premiums? Why or why not?

3. Congratulations! You have just accepted a position as the clinical advisor for a medium-sized health insurance company. You have decided your first priority is to gain control of the costs in your largest insured group, a coal-mining company. Describe the two strategies that you will use and outline at least two initiatives to implement them.

4. You are a member of a healthcare team visiting a developing country in Africa. You are told that healthcare is a right for all people in the country and that the ministry of health is responsible for all care provided. Providers are paid a salary and the ministry runs all the hospitals and clinics. Clinic managers tell you that the ministry usually runs out of money in the eighth or ninth month of the fiscal year. List and discuss the two sources of income you expect providers to have. Which providers do you expect to be the least well paid?

5. The cost of adopting electronic medical records has been shown to be prohibitively high for single-physician and small rural group practices. Discuss the benefits—from the insurer's perspective—of assisting these providers to adopt this technology.

## 3.9. References

Artstein, Z. and Hart, S. 1981. "Law of Large Numbers for Random Sets and Allocation Processes." *Mathematics of Operations Research.* 6 (4): 485–92.

Centers for Medicare and Medicaid Services. "National Health Expenditure Projections 2010–2020." www.cms.gov/NationalHealthExpendData/downloads/proj2010.pdf.

Farber, H. S. 2010. "Job Loss and Decline in Job Security in the United States." In *Labor in the New Economy,* edited by K. S. Abraham, J. R. Spletzer, and M. Harper, 223–62. Chicago: University of Chicago Press.

Follman, T. F. 1962. "Experience Rating vs Community Rating." *Journal of Insurance* 29 (3): 405–15.

Litow, M. 2006. "Medicare versus Private Health Insurance: The Cost of Administration." *Council for Affordable Health Insurance.* 2. Retrieved from www.cahi.org/cahi_contents/resources/pdf/CAHIMedicareTechnicalPaper.pdf.

Telyukov, A., (2012). Provider payment in the healthcare system of the USSR. Personal communication.

# CHAPTER 4

# Healthcare System Strategy and Finance

## 4.1. Chapter Objectives

After completing this chapter you should be able to:

1. Discuss goal setting in the U.S. healthcare system.
2. Define the relationship between goals and financial strategy.
3. Discuss the regulatory challenges that impact goal setting and financial strategy in the U.S. healthcare system.
4. Discuss selected U.S. healthcare system strategic financing dilemmas.

## 4.2. Goal Setting in the U.S. Healthcare System

The healthcare system in the United States was largely a private enterprise until 1965 when President Lyndon B. Johnson signed the Social Security Amendments of 1965 (Social Security, Federal Old Age, Survivors, and Disability Insurance Benefits § 426, 42 U.S.C. § 426 (2012). The legislation authorized federal payment of hospital services and shared payment for physician services for virtually all U.S. citizens 65 years of age and older. Previous to this landmark legislation, the federal government had no significant role in direct payments for healthcare services except for military healthcare (Fetter, 2006). The entry of the federal government into the healthcare market as payer for a large number of civilians opened a new era of healthcare policy and financing in the United States. In 1965 healthcare became a public issue because tax dollars support a large share of the delivery system. A recent review of twenty-five years of public opinion regarding health policy shows that Americans are generally dissatisfied with the current system but satisfied with their own personal healthcare (Blendon *et al.*, 2006). This ambivalence reflects confusion about the purpose of the public healthcare system. Conflicting health-system goals and strategies contribute to this confusion. Despite the major role of the federal government in financing healthcare, the healthcare system in the United States remains fragmented with no unified vision or strategy.

Health-system goals in the United States are inferred rather than specified. There is no public policy document that outlines goals for the entire healthcare system, although the major public systems, for example, military healthcare and Medicare, define their internal goals. The Commonwealth Fund, a private nonprofit organization, has proposed strategic goals and indicators for the entire system (Schoen and How, 2006). Table 4.1 compares these proposed goals with those defined as part of a World Bank discussion paper on general goals for healthcare systems (Schieber, 1997).

Goals are important because they provide the framework for strategic planning. Strategic planning, in turn provides guidance to financial planners because strategy defines investment priorities, cost and revenue projections, and efficiency targets.

In healthcare systems that are dominated by a large public single payer, overall healthcare financing can be targeted to the attainment of specific health-system goals. However, even in well-organized public systems, goal conflicts can be expected. For example, ensuring equity and access to care for all might not be realistic if the system's long-term financial sustainability must also be considered. Achievement of these two potentially conflicting goals would have to be managed through

*TABLE 4.1. Comparative Goals of a Healthcare System.*

| General Goals for Healthcare Systems (Schieber 1997) | Commonwealth Fund U.S. Healthcare System Goals (Schoen and How 2006) |
| --- | --- |
| Improving a population's health status and promoting social well-being | Long, healthy, and productive lives |
| Ensuring equity and access to care | Equity and Access |
| Ensuring macroeconomic and microeconomic efficiency in the use of resources | Efficiency |
| Enhancing clinical effectiveness | (Included in quality goal) |
| Improving quality of care and consumer satisfaction | Quality |
| Assuring the system's long-run financial sustainability | (Included in efficiency goal) |

discussion and compromise, as most stakeholders want both a decent minimum access to care and financial integrity of the system. The same considerations would certainly be true in the case of quality improvement and long-term financial sustainability. Some care quality and consumer satisfaction would have to be sacrificed to ensure financial soundness in the entire system. The extent of this trade-off is usually negotiated among system stakeholders.

Achieving compromise between conflicting health-system goals is a difficult matter. Public single-payer systems are subject to political inertia and large private systems to stockholder and consumer pressures. In the case of blended systems that lack unifying goals, achieving consensus on priorities and compromises needed to define system goals is a difficult if not impossible task.

The Commonwealth Fund's proposal for unified health-system goals illustrates the important role of the private sector in the U.S. healthcare system. Certain public and quasi-public agencies also propose goals for U.S. health-system performance, for example the Healthy People 2020 initiative from Centers for Disease Control and Prevention. All of the proposed goals reflect an attempt to build consensus across a wide array of payers representing various interest groups within the healthcare system. The inevitable conflicts surrounding proposed goals and priorities become difficult to solve across these diverse groups. This complicates the problem of health financing because it is frequently unclear how monetary resources are to be used in healthcare systems given differing focus and priorities of the major stakeholders.

The old adage "he who pays the piper calls the tune" is also true in healthcare financing, as in many other areas of life. As suggested by this aphorism, large payers determine strategy and set financing policy that supports their internal goals. These goals may not be completely congruent with those of other dominant payers in the healthcare market, nor do they match proposed national health goals and financial priorities. Evidence for this disconnect is presented in a recent study of the needs of the private sector for relevant health services research to support their organizational goals (Schur *et al.*, 2009). The study finds almost no congruence between health services research supported by public-sector funders and the information needs of private-sector health systems to plan and finance care for their clients.

## 4.3. The Relationship between Goals and Financial Strategy

In the private sector, strategic planning provides a guide for financial managers on how to commit a firm's financial resources to achieve corporate goals. Myers (1984) suggests that the financial part of the enterprise is subordinate to the organizational strategy defined for the firm. Certainly, financial managers participate in corporate goal setting, but they do not independently determine corporate goals. Financial managers use tools of finance such as capital asset planning and budgeting to maximize achievement of previously defined corporate goals. Financial tools are also used to evaluate the firm's financial efficiency and effectiveness and to measure financial performance in the context of corporate goals. This linkage between goals, strategic planning, and financial management is important to the success of the firm. Organizational research shows that a strong linkage between corporate strategic planning and financial management correlates with competitive advantage in the market (Teece, Pisano, and Shuen, 1997).

The public sector also tries to link system goals and financial management. Williams (2004) provides a review of the historical development of performance-based budgeting in the United States. Williams suggests that the linkages between the strategic goals for government spending, public budgets, and performance measurements of goal attainment emerged at the start of the twentieth century and continue to the present day. At the federal and state levels, linkages between the public-sector budget and the government's performance against stated objectives are mandated by government agencies and their political directors. A recent review of the public-budgeting process at the state level found that 39 states also have some level of performance-based budgeting linking government spending with defined goals within their administrative codes (Rubin and Willoughby, 2011).

This goal-oriented process is also in place at the federal level. However, the linkages between the strategic direction articulated by the executive branch and the allocation of funds by means of a budget negotiated with Congress are often not completely congruent (Joyce, 2011). Unlike the private sector, the public budget is judged not only by attainment of stated goals but also by the acceptability of the goals themselves to elected officials in Congress. This creates a situation in which financial management of healthcare services in the public sector is evaluated against the double standard of performance against stated goals and the political acceptability of the defined healthcare goals. For example, the 2010 Patient Protection and Affordable Care Act (U.S. Code 2010, PL 111-148, 124 Stat 119) contains a mandate that requires every citizen to purchase health insurance or pay a penalty. This is an actuarially sound strategy to increase the participation of the healthy in the insurance market to ensure against adverse selection and maintain affordable group insurance rates. However, this requirement was challenged in the courts as a violation of the federalist principle. In this example it can be seen that the public-sector goal to maintain affordable health-insurance premiums for all and decrease the number of uninsured individuals in the United States was presented as unconstitutional by political opponents of the reform architects. The technically correct solution to the problem may suffer a setback on considerations of constitutional unacceptability. Political differences such as those seen in this example hamper the potential effectiveness of public-sector strategic planning in healthcare.

Public-sector systems may not be able to achieve optimal efficiency in healthcare due to the political nature of the system in which they operate. In a democratic system political accountability to the electorate is a deeply held value that cannot be set aside. The shared social compact, then, is an important mediator in democratically governed public-sector systems. This implies that development of shared societal agreements on desired system priorities, level of acceptable public expense, and role and relationship of the system to individual and public health are essential if the system is to function effectively within the political context.

## 4.4.  Goals, Strategy, and Finance in the U.S. Healthcare System

The previous discussion shows how complex determining the strategic objectives that guide resource allocation can be in the U.S. healthcare system. For example, should public resources be provided to maximize goals related to public health or goals related to individual healthcare? Since 1965, the federal government has assumed responsibility for delivering personal healthcare to a significant number of U.S. citizens through Medicare and Medicaid. Yet we know from research into the determinants of health that the marginal contribution that medical care makes to population health is small (Fuchs, 1986, 272–299). However, for an individual who is in poor health, healthcare is a vital resource that can easily make the difference between life and death. The conflict between using public funds to increase the health of the entire population or to provide essential personal healthcare to individuals who require it has become a debate in healthcare strategic planning and finance.

Immunization policy is an example of this dilemma. There is excellent scientific support for the cost-effectiveness of basic vaccines in increasing the health of the population. The basic childhood vaccines as well as influenza and pneumococcal vaccines for adults increase health at a moderate cost. Yet research shows that 15 percent of children and 30 percent of adults are enrolled in private health plans that do not provide coverage for these vaccines (Davis and Fant, 2005). These same plans likely provide basic hospital and physician benefits for both children and adults, and set their premiums based on the likelihood that such services might be required. The strategic objective for these health plans, as reflected in their coverage choices, is not preventive services but rather individual healthcare in the event of an illness.

The strategic decision not to provide vaccine coverage despite the proven health benefits can be explained by examining the payer's priorities. The payer may know that the long-term investment in vaccine coverage is not profitable because beneficiaries are not enrolled in the plan long enough to benefit the organization. If beneficiary turnover is high, there is no cost recovery from vaccinations or other forms of prevention. Some payers do not provide these services unless they are mandated by the purchaser or by insurance regulators because they do not benefit from the reduced cost of care in the event of a vaccine-preventable disease.

Even if goals are agreed, accomplishing them is problematic. In the public sector, for example, the federal budget process is a synthesis of "bottom-up" budgetary requests made by agencies and "top-down" prioritization in response to the strategic and political vision of the administration. Federal agencies are focused on activity areas such as health, environmental protection, commerce, social welfare, or international assistance, and they request funding for their internal missions without regard for crossover with other agencies working on similar strategic goals. The goal of improving public health depends not only on funding the Department of Health and Human Services but also on funding many other agencies that affect population health. The Environmental Protection Agency, for example, ensures clean air and water; the Department of Education ensures basic education; and the Department of State regulates international travel and immigration to the United States. Maximizing population health involves all of these agencies and may require increasing the funding of one at the expense of another.

In a debate about resource allocation, the urgent needs of individuals requiring personal healthcare services create competition for scarce public funds that could also be used to support population health. Within personal healthcare, resource competition takes place between preventive and curative care. According to a 2011 study, preventive services account for 6 percent of all public spending on personal healthcare while care of chronic and acute illness and trauma account for the remaining 94 percent. (Conway *et al.*, 2011).

The political dimension of these allocation dilemmas is important because each individual who needs healthcare is also a voter. As individual healthcare paid for with public funds expands, so does the political support for these programs at the expense of public-health programs without such a clearly defined constituency. As the share of the elderly in the nation's population grows, so does support for curative care at the expense of prevention programs.

The private sector financing problem is less complex because a private firm is not concerned with public priorities. Each healthcare firm defines its financial strategy to maximize its performance against pre-defined strategic goals. Each organization wants to maximize its return on investment, either to serve its owners or stockholders, in the case of for-profit companies, or, with nonprofits, to fund its charitable activities. These companies are not concerned with the overall health of the population; rather they are concerned with production of the services or products for which they bill. Regulators can mandate certain services within the private healthcare organization's strategic scope, for example immunization services. However, regulators cannot completely change the strategic objectives of the healthcare organization; regulators can only influence how these objectives are achieved.

An excellent example of this dynamic between regulators and providers is the implementation of the diagnosis-related groups (DRGs) to reimburse hospitals for services to Medicare beneficiaries. The federal government introduced the DRG-based rate schedule in 1984. The rates were established per discharged patient and based on the bundle of services provided for a specific diagnosis, not on each item of service provided. DRG rates are estimated based on a DRG-specific length of stay, sufficient to treat an average case in the DRG. If a hospital used more days to provide care, it incurred a financial loss. Conversely, if the hospital delivered care in less time, reimbursement was likely to exceed cost, and the hospital stood to benefit financially. Hospitals quickly learned how to deliver care more efficiently, and the average length of stay in an acute care hospital decreased significantly. The decrease in average length of stay (ALOS) was so significant that it compensated for the increased admissions that occurred due to the increase in number of Medicare beneficiaries over the period depicted in Figure 4.1. This resulted in a steady decrease in patient days (ALOS × Admissions) despite an increase in Medicare enrollees.

However, as shown in Figure 4.2, the trend in the aggregate cost for acute care under Medicare over the same period shows a steady increase in hospital costs despite decreased utilization.

These data illustrate the focus that hospital executives have on maximizing financial results for their institutions despite regulatory strategies that attempt to increase efficiency and control costs. The factors that drove this steady increase in cost despite a steady decrease in utilization are directly attributable to careful financial management that maximizes reimbursement for every Medicare stay. A recent working paper from the National Bureau of Economic Research (Dafney, 2003)

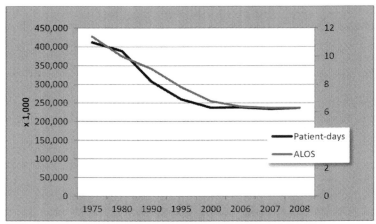

***FIGURE 4.1.*** *Trends in Patient Days (on the left vertical scale) and Average Length of Stay (on the right vertical scale) in U.S. Hospitals 1975–2008. Source: Centers for Disease Control and Prevention.*

confirms that hospital financial managers employ sophisticated coding strategies to classify their patients into more expensive DRGs and maximize Medicare reimbursement. These strategies result in increased revenue despite considerable efficiency gains in hospital service delivery.

The reviewed examples illustrate the role of the regulator in influencing strategic decisions and the adaptive responses of corporate managers that maximize financial outcomes under changed compliance rules.

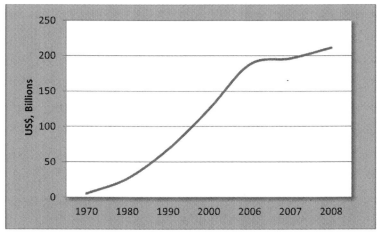

***FIGURE 4.2.*** *Medicare U.S. Hospital Costs 1970–2008. Source: Centers for Disease Control and Prevention.*

## 4.5.  Strategic Dilemmas in U.S. Healthcare

Three major strategic dilemmas facing the U.S. healthcare system are: (1) whether to support allocation of public resources to personal healthcare, (2) whether to keep up access to expensive healthcare technologies and pharmaceuticals, and (3) whether to establish mandatory participation of the individual in a group insurance system. There are no clear answers to these dilemmas, and healthcare providers need to consider carefully their role and position regarding these issues.

Allocation of public resources for personal healthcare is a pressing issue given the relentlessly growing demand for public funding to pay for these services. As shown in Figure 4.3, federal spending on health is projected to be 30 percent of the entire federal budget by 2016.

As we have seen in our previous discussions, the largest portion of these federal outlays are for personal healthcare services that are supported through Medicare, Medicaid, military healthcare, and health insurance for federal workers. The estimates in Figure 4.3 may underestimate the level of funds required, but even this relatively conservative estimate shows the magnitude of growth in public spending for healthcare. The source of funds for these programs is either current tax receipts, or when this revenue is insufficient, government debt. The size of the current government debt has created a vigorous debate in U.S.

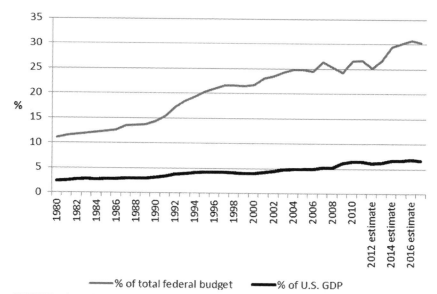

*FIGURE 4.3.  Federal Spending on Health as a Percent of Federal Budget and GDP. Source: Office of Management and Budget.*

Congress regarding the need for fiscal constraint in order to decrease deficit spending and lower the cost of government borrowing. As the public commitment to pay for personal healthcare services grows, it increasingly is at odds with the demand for fiscal restraint. Containing public spending on personal health becomes an urgent task.

There are limited ways to achieve this reduction in public spending. Certainly eliminating waste, fraud, and abuse is extremely important, but these measures are not expected to result in enough savings. They have to be supported by reduced programmatic commitments, which implies decreasing the number of individuals eligible for benefits, restricting the benefits themselves, or both. Healthcare providers can expect to be increasingly involved in these discussions as public sector programs look for ways to limit public spending.

A further complication of this debate is the extent to which public money should be spent for healthcare services as opposed to initiatives to preserve and enhance the health of the population. This discussion centers on the consumption-or-investment dilemma. Prevention programs require an investment in health-enhancing programs to avoid the need for healthcare spending later. Delivery of acute care services to individuals, particularly those who are chronically ill, represents consumption that is not likely to improve the population's health. The feasibility of using large amounts of public funds to subsidize consumption of care by the elderly rather than investing public funds in the health of the young merits careful analysis and discussion regarding the purpose of government and the need for generational equity.

Access to expensive technology and pharmaceuticals is an ongoing debate, particularly for programs funded by the public sector. Soumerai (2004) provides an insightful discussion of the benefits and risks of decreasing access to costly pharmaceuticals in the Medicaid program. This discussion highlights the typical dilemmas faced by payers, providers, and consumers when policies designed to limit access to costly technologies and drugs are considered. For example, forcing providers to switch to less costly generic drugs does result in significant savings, although there are increased costs in physician utilization as chronically ill individuals with complex medication regimens make the change to generic dosing regimens. In systems that are underserved, these increased provider visits may be delayed or impossible, which in turn may result in increased morbidity or mortality for the chronically ill. The trade-off considerations necessary in these situations are complex and poorly understood. For example, decreasing access to mammograms in younger women is undoubtedly cost-effective for the majority of women. However, determining whether a woman should be an exception to the under-fifty mammogram policy assumes a level of health literacy, and provider access that may not be uniformly present. Certainly, further research is needed to compare these risks with the known risks of false positives and routine mammography costs in the general population of women under fifty. Providers need to be engaged in these areas of research to ensure that the evidence needed to make responsible decisions regarding limitation on technology and pharmaceuticals is provided.

Providers need to be engaged in these areas of research to help provide evidence for responsible decisions on whether/how to limit the use of technology and pharmaceuticals. One of the primary considerations is the requirement that healthy individuals who do not expect major health expenses purchase group health insurance in order to provide a subsidy for individuals who are sick. The general argument is that there is no certainty that any given individual will not require healthcare services. Accidents or unexpected illness can happen to anyone, and health insurance is needed to protect every individual from these catastrophic expenses. Additionally, the social compact that mandates availability of lifesaving healthcare services to everyone in need regardless of ability to pay results in financial liabilities for the providers of these essential services. These liabilities must be paid, and the source of payment is an additional charge to the insured users of acute services, a hidden sickness tax. It is levied on the patients or third-party payers to reimburse providers for uncompensated emergency services. Insurers are increasingly unwilling to pay these additional charges, and public payers do not pay them since they base their payments on the cost of care delivered to beneficiaries rather than the charges determined by the provider. Thus the cost of uncompensated care is shifted to the privately insured population who are increasingly unwilling to pay full charges. Analysts suggest that the only way out of this "death-spiral" trend is to mandate health insurance coverage for every individual. Arguably, this mandate violates the deeply held value in U.S. society for autonomy. Certainly, individuals may be required to pay tax when they purchase commodities, and there are also mandatory insurance requirements at the state level for drivers, owners of property, and business owners. However, the requirement to purchase health insurance is not limited to a particular category of individuals. The universal requirement to purchase insurance by virtue of U.S. citizenship is unprecedented and may not be possible without a Constitutional amendment. Providers need to increase their understanding of this fundamental dilemma faced by U.S. society and engage in public debate regarding feasible solutions. The role of tax policy, the effectiveness of state-level programs, and provider social responsibility are all aspects of this problem that need more research, analysis, and discussion.

## 4.6. Concept Checkout

Be sure you understand the following concepts before you begin the discussion questions:

- Goal setting in public and private health systems
- Relationship of goals, strategic planning, and financial strategy
- Regulatory impact on strategic planning
- Health and healthcare in public and private sector payment systems
- Allocation of public resources to pay for individual healthcare
- Access to expensive technology and drugs
- Individual mandate to purchase health insurance

## 4.7. Discussion Questions

1. Describe the essential difference between goal setting in public and private health-insurance systems.
2. Explain the relationship between goals, strategic objectives, and financial strategy using an example from either public or private health-insurance organizations.
3. Debate at least one potential strategic dilemma confronting a health insurer. Provide at least one tentative solution to resolve the dilemma.
4. Differentiate the roles of the public-sector regulator and the private-sector strategic planner in immunization policy and service delivery.
5. Outline a provider position paper in response to one of the three strategic dilemmas discussed in this chapter. Your position paper outline may be focused at either the state or federal level. The outline may represent your personal view as a provider or the view of a provider organization.

## 4.8. References

Blendon, R. J., M. Brodie, J. M. Benson, D. E. Altman, T. Buhr. 2006. "American's View of Healthcare Quality." *Milbank Quarterly* 84:4: 623–57.

Conway, P., K. Goodrich, S. Machlin, B. Sasse, J. Cohen. 2011. "Patient-Centered Care Categorization of U.S. Health-Care Expenditures." *Health Services Research* 46 (2): 479–90.

Dafney, L. S. 2003. "How Do Hospitals Respond to Price Changes?" *NBER Working Paper Series* Working Paper 9972: NBER 1–49.

Davis, M., K. Fant. 2005. "Coverage of Vaccines in Private Health Plans: What Does the Public Prefer?" *Health Affairs* 24 (3): 770–79.

Fetter, B. 2006. "The Origins and Elaborations of the National Health Accounts, 1920–1966." *Healthcare Financing Review* 28 (1): 53–67.

Fuchs, V. 1986. *The Health Economy.* Cambridge, Mass: Harvard University Press.

Joyce, P. G. 2011. "The Obama Administration and PBB: Building on the Legacy of Federal PBB." *Public Administration Review* 71 (3): 356–67.

Myers, S. 1984. "Finance Theory and Financial Strategy." *Interfaces* 14 (1): 126–37.

Rubin, M. and K. Willoughby. 2011. "Measuring Government Performance: The Intersection of Strategic Planning and Performance Budgeting." *Transatlantic Dialogue Conference Proceedings.*

Schieber, G., and A. Maeda. 1997. "Curmudgeon's Guide to Financing Health Care in Developing Countries." *Innovations in Health Care Financing: Proceedings of a World Bank Conference,* World Bank Discussion Paper, No 365.

Schoen, C. and S. K. How. 2006. "U.S. Health System Performance: A National Scorecard." *The Commonwealth Fund.* www.commonwealthfund.org/Publications/In-the-Literature/2006/Sep/U-S--Health-System-Performance--A-National-Scorecard.aspx.

Schur, C., M. Burk, L. Silver, J. Yeglan, and M. O'Grady. 2009. "Connecting the Ivory Tower to Main Street: Setting Research Priorities for Real World Impact." *Health Affairs* 28 (5): 886–99.

Social Security, Federal Old Age, Survivors, and Disability Insurance Benefits § 426, 42 U.S.C. § 426 (2010)

Social Security, Federal Old Age, Survivors, and Disability Insurance Benefits § 426, 42 U.S.C. § 426 (2012).

Teece, D. J., G. Pisano, and A. Shuen. 1997. "Dynamic Capabilities and Strategic Management." *Strategic Management Journal* 18 (7): 509–33.

U.S. Office of Management and Budget. Omnibus Budget. www.whitehouse.gov/omb/budget/Historicals.

Williams, D. W. 2004. "Performance Measurement and Performance Budgeting in the United States in the 1950s and 1960s." *Proceedings of the Conference of the European Group of Public Administration.* http://webh01.ua.ac.be/pubsector/ljubljana/Williams_paper.pdf.

# The Prisoner's Dilemma

*You should not attempt this case until you have completed Chapters 1 through 4 in your textbook.*

*The facts in the case:*

You have been appointed as the state commissioner for prison health care. Your scope of responsibility includes management of the acute and ambulatory care system for the state prison population of 13,000. Here are a few facts about this population:

- Approximately 21,000 offenders are admitted for incarceration and 21,000 released each year.
- 60 percent are sentenced to serve more than one year.
- 10 percent are sentenced to less than one year.
- 30 percent are offenders in detention status.
- Prison is for those serving one or more years.
- Jail is for those serving less than a year or for those being detained.
- The average length of stay for the detention population is 30 days.
- The average length of stay for the jailed population is 54 days.
- The average length of stay for the prison population is 20.7 months.

The benefits that you provide to this population are:

- Medical services
- Nursing services
- Mental health services
- Dental services
- Pharmacy services

- Specialty consultation
- Female healthcare services
- Utilization review services
- Substance abuse treatment
- Inpatient hospital services

The cost summary for the past year is shown in Table CS2.1.

The services are provided by a contracted managed-care organization that provides stipulated benefits. The cost of services are reflected in the negotiated contract amount in line 1. All items marked with an asterisk are your overhead costs. The last two line-items may be considered preventive costs that are not covered by the managed care contract, but are directly provided by your department to prisoners, not to those in detention or the jailed population staying less than one year.

The demographics of the prison population (those serving more than 1 year) show that 80 percent of them are male and 20 percent are female. Prisoners over age 55 represent 7 percent of the male and 5 percent of the female population. The median age of the prisoners is 32. The majority of the prisoners are from households at or below the poverty line, and 70 percent are from minority groups. The average level of education across the inmate population is 10 or fewer years of formal education, 40 percent of the prison population is estimated to be functionally illiterate. Twenty percent of the prisoners are HIV positive and 7 percent have a history of TB. Drugs and other substance abuse are

TABLE CS2.1. Annual Health Services Expenditures.

| Item | Cost |
| --- | --- |
| Negotiated Contract | $38,039,831 |
| Other related medical costs not covered by negotiated contract | $2,800,000 |
| *Current correctional health staff positions (including other employee costs) | $620,300 |
| *Correctional health office equipment | $50,000 |
| *Travel and  training for correctional health staff | $10,000 |
| *Miscellaneous/auditing by correctional health staff | $25,000 |
| *Contractual services related to correctional health department external to prisoner's health | $150,000 |
| *Operating costs of the correctional health department | $15,000 |
| *Nonoperational correctional health department costs | $2,800,000 |
| *Training/consultant costs for correctional health department | $750,000 |
| Immunizations provided to prisoners | $1,150,000 |
| Monitor costs for prisoners | $90,000 |
| Total costs | $46,500,131 |

problems for 45 percent of the population, although those with active dependency are limited to 20 percent of the inmate population.

*The problem:*

You have been asked to reduce healthcare spending in the population because the state budget has been cut by 12 percent, and further cuts are expected. The majority of costs are in the prison population (those staying more than one year). Your analysis should focus on this population. The managed-care organization that holds the contract has informed you that it is expecting a price increase in the next fiscal year and that it will not be able to bid on the next managed care contract unless the amount is increased at least 5 percent above the current level. You are considering taking the contract in-house and want to assess carefully the ramifications of this decision.

Your case analysis should answer the following questions:

1. What are the current total administrative costs for the Department of Prison Health, and what is the per-prisoner cost of medical care?
2. Given the prisoner demographics and based on your research, what type of healthcare costs and what cost distribution might you expect?
3. Suggest at least three strategies to decrease the amount of loss given the current cost data shown in Table CS2.1. Include in your suggestions an assessment of the feasibility and possible intended and unintended outcomes of each loss-reduction strategy you recommend.
4. Suggest at least three strategies to decrease the probability that financial loss will occur in this population based on your research and assessment of prisoner healthcare costs. Include an analysis of the feasibility and potential outcomes of each recommended strategy.
5. Discuss at least two potential effects on your prison health costs if universal health insurance were to be mandated for all residents of your state. Provide a rationale for each effect you identify.

You may make reasonable assumptions about the burden and distribution of disease in this population. Please conduct some research on prisoner health in order to make these assumptions. Remember that states may mandate coverage for the prison population in a variety of ways. For example, the state may consider including prisoners in the health-insurance exchange pool and ask that the Department of Corrections assume the premium cost during the time that the prisoner is incarcerated. Remember also that this is a state prison system, not a federal system. The considerations are quite different at the state level because prison stays are shorter, and the state makes both Medicaid and prison health policy. One of the major problems for prisoners is continuity of care after release. This is a particular problem when prisoners must transition from a prison healthcare system to a private insurance system. Consider this problem as you make your recommendations.

# Section 3

# Financial Management in Healthcare Markets

## 5.1. Chapter Objectives

After completing the chapter you should be able to:

1. Discuss the basic financial incentives in the U.S. healthcare market.
2. Define healthcare financial management strategies as a response to market incentives.
3. Explain the linkage between healthcare financial management and operations management.
4. Define the major parts of an organizational financial plan.

## 5.2. Financial Incentives in the U.S. Healthcare Market

This chapter links the macro-finance concepts in the preceding four chapters with the financial strategies, tools, and actions that enable competent financial management of a primary care practice. Excellence in financial management requires the use of financial information to achieve strategic goals and organizational survival. That is why healthcare financial managers require an understanding of internal organizational strategy, good financial management practice, and the economic environment surrounding the healthcare organization.

Healthcare organizations in the United States operate in a highly regulated environment composed of public and private payers that employ market incentives to achieve results. Healthcare financial managers need to understand the basic principles that define a competitive market and have detailed knowledge of the market regulatory environment.

We have seen that the two essential actors in a market-based economy are consumers and firms. These actors meet and exchange resources through a market. A market is composed of firms and individuals (consumers) that are in touch with each other to buy or sell some good (Mansfield, 1980). Economic theory suggests that that the consumer is assured of the widest availability of goods at the lowest possible price under conditions of perfect market competition. We know that perfect competition is a theoretical concept that cannot be completely operationalized; however, understanding the theoretical characteristics of an efficient competitive market provides a basis for understanding the deviations in healthcare markets (Austin and Hungerford, 2009). In theory, a perfectly competitive market has:

"1) many buyers and sellers—each participant is small in relation to the market and cannot affect the price through its own actions;
2) neither consumption nor production generates spillover benefits or costs;
3) free entry and exit from the market—new firms can open up shop and existing firms can costlessly leave the market as conditions change;
4) symmetric information—all market participants know the same things so that no one has an informational advantage over others;
5) no transaction costs—the buyers and sellers incur no additional cost in making the transaction, and the complexity of decisions has no effect on choices;
6) firms maximize profits and consumers maximize well-being."
(Austin and Hungerford 2009)

We can see that the healthcare market has numerous characteristics that deviate from an open competitive market. For example, the healthcare market is distorted by a lack of information on the part of consumers, high market entry costs for suppliers of healthcare services, a regulated complex environment that results in significant transactions costs, and many nonprofit healthcare delivery firms are given tax advantages to maximize service volume rather than profit. All of these competitive market distortions must be considered in financial planning. Additionally, the U.S. healthcare market has undergone major changes since Medicare and Medicaid legislation was enacted. These changes are due not only to the aging of the U.S. population but also to the regulatory power of the public payers that can create market incentives. State and federal governments also create legislation and regulation that impacts the healthcare market. Access to information has also changed markedly over the past forty years. The increased availability of information available to payers and the public has enriched the understanding of healthcare delivery and expanded the community standard that guides decisions on the delivery of care.

Four major market incentives are active in the U.S. healthcare market today: process safety, process efficiency, optimal outcomes of care, and overall cost effectiveness of care (Barone, 2008). This incentive structure suggests that providers must always consider patient safety in addition to efficient production of care since payers, regulators, and the courts will penalize unsafe provision of care regardless of efficiency. This means that the financial manager needs to evaluate practice costs in the context of safety. Decisions such as the selection of practice supplies, equipment, and personnel cannot be predicated only on cost-minimization principles because low costs may reflect unwarranted compromises in safety. For example, a practice may choose to employ unlicensed personnel to handle patient flow and support, or the practice may expend additional funds to hire licensed nurses for the same purpose. The parameters that guide this decision are not only salary savings but also the additional training and knowledge that licensed personnel bring to patient management. Such decisions require information systems that enable careful analysis of patient acuity, practice requirements, and the prevailing community standard to assure an acceptable level of safety and cost.

Outcomes of care have always been a major consideration for patients as well as for providers. However, it has not always been possible to access sufficient data to conduct careful comparisons of patient-care outcomes. The advent of large clinical datasets and increased computer capability has greatly enhanced the scope and power of outcomes assessment. Today payers and patients expect clinicians to be current with the best evidence on clinical outcomes and to select therapies accordingly. In an early discussion of clinical outcomes, Zimmerman and Daley (1997) point out six outcome considerations: quality, cost-effectiveness, access, patient satisfaction, and resource use. These considerations suggest that it is important to weigh aggregate cost-effectiveness not only against safety but also in consideration of individual patient concerns. For example, recent recommendations regarding the use of mammography in young women with no risk factors for breast cancer (U.S. Preventative Services Task Force, 2009) are focused on the most efficient use of expensive medical resources. Breast cancer in young women is a rare occurrence, and detecting it exposes women to the costs and potential harms of false positive findings. However, for the rare young woman who actually has invasive breast cancer, the fact that routine mammography is the most cost-effective solution for society is not as important as early detection of the condition. In this case, the cost-effective choice that benefits society does little to benefit the young woman with invasive breast cancer. Clinicians and financial managers need to consider the issue of clinical efficacy and cost-effectiveness in the context of individual patient welfare and make careful therapeutic choices. In some cases, the patient's wishes, the clinical recommendation, and the payers' policies may not be congruent, forcing complex clinical choices. This type of dilemma illustrates the complexity of the healthcare market because the recipient of care seldom pays its entire cost. It often happens that the market incentives that define the payer's decisions do not align completely with the incentives that define the patient's decisions. The healthcare provider tries to maximize the outcome for the patient as well as assuring acceptable financial returns on the process of care. Good communication, adequate information, and careful negotiation are required among patient, provider, and payer to respond adequately to healthcare market incentives and to satisfy the consumer's needs.

Healthcare organizations also pursue strategic goals in a regulatory environment that does not consider the optimal financial performance of individual firms as a primary goal. Instead, the goal of maximizing access to healthcare services, even for those who cannot pay, is considered more important than preserving a competitive market that allows firms to maximize profits and benefit shareholders. The resulting trade-off is in the efficient volume maximization. The latter is offered to, and frequently accepted by providers as a basic market incentive under public and private provider contracts.

Healthcare regulation is generally considered to be the responsibility of the state rather than the federal government. The state licenses healthcare providers and facilities and regulates health insurers that operate within the state. The state' role in controlling access to the healthcare market is extremely important, and financial managers need to be aware of state regulations that shape market entry and continued participation in the market.

However, once a provider is able to enter the market, the entity that actually pays for healthcare services assumes a central role. Figure 5.1 shows the share of healthcare expenditures assumed by the four categories of payers (sponsors). The National Health Expenditure Accounts defines sponsors as the entity ultimately responsible for paying the healthcare bill. The amount of spending by households includes its share of health insurance co-payments; the amount spent by businesses on premiums for its employees is categorized under private enterprise.

Payers control provider participation in their segment of the market. For example, the federally funded program for the elderly, Medicare, requires that providers be enrolled in the Medicare program before they can bill for the services they provide. This is also true for many private insurers that require providers to qualify to become a preferred network

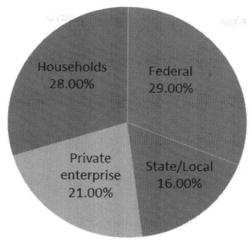

**FIGURE 5.1.** *Share of Health Spending By Sponsor, 2010. Source: Centers for Medicare and Medicaid Services.*

provider. Consumers who select out-of-network providers may do so but are discouraged by higher co-payments for selecting such a provider.

### 5.3. Healthcare Financial Management Strategies as a Response to Market Incentives

A financial manager must, therefore, understand the incentives created by the regulatory requirements for market entry on two levels: (1) the primary entry to the market, which is controlled by the state through licensure of providers and facilities, and (2) entries to segments of the market controlled by third-party payers.

A healthcare organization makes a strategic decision about market entry when it decides what type of services it will offer, which networks it will join, and what type of third-party payment it will accept. Once those decisions are made, the financial manager must understand the regulatory conditions the payer has defined for market participation. These include the requirements for provider enrollment and the billing and reimbursement policies. The healthcare organization's strategic management team should carefully examine these reimbursement policies because they define market incentives that shape organizational financial strategy and market behavior of the organization.

In order to negotiate viable contracts, providers need to conduct a reimbursement analysis that examines the incentives inherent in the payer's reimbursement policies. A general outline of such an analysis is shown in Figure 5.2.

### Reimbursement Analysis

A reimbursement analysis should gather information from each prospective payer in the following areas:

What is the beneficiary base?

Information should be provided on the number of covered beneficiaries the provider can expect. In the case of public payers such as Medicare and Medicaid, population data may be required as well as data on other providers in the region. It is also important to understand the restrictions on switching from one primary care provider to another once the beneficiary enrolls.

What services are reimbursed?

The covered services and exclusions for the beneficiaries should be clearly defined. If there are second-opinion requirements, waiting periods, or other qualifying events, they need to be clearly stipulated. The procedures for appeal of denied reimbursement also need to be clearly understood. Particular attention should be paid to clinical services such as patient education, counseling, and consultation. Many payers reimburse for these services, but providers do not always know that they can recover payment. All billable services should be clearly understood.

How is reimbursement requested and received?

Provider enrollment requirements, billing formats and coding, information system linkages and requirements, arrangements for payment transmittal, and the basis for reimbursement requests should all be defined. For example, if a fee schedule is the basis for reimbursement, the provider needs to understand if any deviation from this schedule will be allowed. If the basis for reimbursement is cost or discounted cost, then the documentation required to establish the cost base needs to be clear, as does the effective period for the cost schedule.

What is the payer's incentive and penalty structure?

In addition to payments for services, many payers make bonus payments if service or quality targets are achieved. Conditions for these bonus payments and penalties for undesired events should be clear.

Who qualifies for payment?

Group practices frequently comprise physicians, advanced practice nurses, and other health professionals such as clinical psychologists, physical therapists, or registered dietitians. A reimbursement analysis should clearly define who may bill directly for services and who must bill under another professional's billing authorization. The services that are billable under each professional's billing authorization also need to be clear. The time required and the procedures for credentialing a provider to enable him or her to bill should also be clearly understood.

*FIGURE 5.2. Reimbursement Analysis.*

The outlined reimbursement analysis uses published reimbursement policies from the public payers or information requested from a prospective private payer. This analysis is a critical input for contract negotiation before a provider agreement is signed. Individualized contract negotiation with public payers is difficult because all providers who accept public payment are generally treated in a similar way. However, a reimbursement analysis is still important since it will inform provider practice and financial policies once the decision is made to accept either Medicare or Medicaid contracts.

## 5.4. The Linkage between Healthcare Financial Management and Operations Management

In general the financial management plan involves three major analytic areas: market entry and participation; reimbursement and revenue planning; and financial operations management. The first two areas require a clear understanding of external actors: the regulators and payers previously discussed. The final analytic area, financial operations management, is focused on the internal activities of the provider organization. The financial management skills presented in the last half of this textbook support this important area.

Financial managers provide information to operations managers to enable them to understand resource use in the context of their operational objectives. Financial managers also provide information that is critical to the evaluation of operations. Operations managers need to understand the cost-benefit relationship of their strategies as well as the impact of decisions on the organization's revenue. Finally, managers consider the operational resource use that impacts quality and safety in the context of both consumer preference and regulatory guidance. As in the case of mammograms for young women, there is a financial, operational, and consumer preference dimension inherent in most quality and safety decisions made in healthcare organizations. Information provided by the financial manager supports informed decisions in this and all areas of operations management.

Information is the basic link between financial and operations management. Financial analysis generally focuses on the firm's financial performance by analyzing revenue, expenses, and reimbursement. Operating analysis focuses on factors such as patient visits, case-mix, and use of ancillary services. The financial manager typically organizes reports to operations managers on a periodic basis. Depending on the volatility of the operation, such reporting can be daily, weekly, or monthly.

Enterprise resource planning information systems introduce the possibility of real-time links between financial and operations management. These systems require significant start-up planning, costly implementation, and detailed input data. A recent industry analysis of these integrated systems shows that they are not yet an optimal answer to the need for integrated financial and operations data in healthcare (KLAS, 2010). However, the evolution of the healthcare market suggests that the need for timely, accurate, and integrated financial and operations data drives developers to produce better solutions and provide integrated platforms to support primary as well as acute care. At this point the financial information available to operations should be as accurate, useful, and timely as possible. Financial reports should be easy for the operations manager to understand and provide information needed to adjust operational strategy as quickly as possible to optimize financial and strategic goals.

## 5.5.  The Organizational Financial Plan

Large organizations typically have long-term and short-term financial plans. Long-term plans focus on how the organization will find the financial resources to remain in business over the long-term planning horizon, typically five to seven years. This type of planning requires a thorough understanding of market trends and financing strategies available to the firm. For example, firms that are publically owned can plan stock offerings that are timed to meet the firm's capital requirements. The firm can consider a mixture of equity (stock) and debt (bonds) to provide needed capital for expansion or acquisition of technology. Long-term financial planning for healthcare organizations is challenging due to the nature of the market. We have seen that almost half of the health spending in the U.S. market is controlled by federal, state, or local governments. This means that political, regulatory, and demographic trends have a great influence on revenue expectations. These revenue expectations influence the extent to which healthcare providers need to consider other sources of capital to support their technology-intensive operations. Forecasting models that can predict the effect of these influences on the healthcare market are essential for long-term financial planning.

Short-term financial planning is much more concerned with immediate influences on income and expenses. Short-term financial plans typically start with the organization's annual budget. After the budget is defined, the actual financial performance of the organization is compared to the budget projected for the period. The extent to which the actual performance varies from the projected revenue and expenses is reviewed. Based on this review, operational changes are made to ensure that the organization meets its short-term financial goals. The main reports that are used in short-term financial planning are the budget and the variance report, which focuses on variances from the budget in revenue and expense. Variance reports are typically broken down by department so that each operational manager is aware of departmental performance against projections. The chapters that follow provide the information necessary to develop financial plans for a healthcare organization and measure the actual performance against the plan.

## 5.6. Concept Checkout

Be sure you understand the following concepts before you begin the discussion questions:

- Free-market characteristics
- Healthcare market incentives
- Market entry requirements
- Reimbursement analysis
- Information as the critical link between finance and operations
- Long-term financial planning
- Short-term financial planning

## 5.7. Discussion Questions

1. Describe the characteristics of a perfectly competitive market and give one actual example of how healthcare markets differ from those that are perfectly competitive.
2. Define each of the four main healthcare market incentives and give a recent actual example of each incentive from the context of the payer and the provider.
3. Select one major public or private payer for healthcare services and list all the conditions that the primary care provider must meet to qualify for reimbursement.
4. List and define all the components that should be included in a reimbursement analysis from the perspective of a primary healthcare provider. Give one actual or theoretical example of each component.
5. Define the information required to understand the cost of a routine primary healthcare visit.
6. Select either long- or short-term financial planning as your focus, give one real-world example of a planning strategy used in your focus area, and discuss the information that would be needed to evaluate success or failure of the strategy.

## 5.8. References

Austin, D. A., and T. L. Hungerford. 2009. "The Market Structure of the Health Insurance Industry." *Congressional Research Service Report* R40834. www.fas.org/sgp/crs/misc/R40834.pdf.

Barone, D. 2008. "Time-to-Adoption: Reimbursement as a Marketing Strategy." Retrieved from www.bmtadvisors.com/docs/%27Time%20to%20Adoption%27%20-%20Reimbursement%20as%20a%20Marketing%20Strategy%20Paradigm.pdf.

Centers for Medicare and Medicaid Services. "National Health Expenditure 2010 Highlights." www.cms.gov/Research-Statistics-Data-and-Systems/Statistics-Trends-and-Reports/NationalHealthExpendData/downloads/sponsors.pdf.

Zimmerman, D. and J. Daley. 1997. "Using Outcomes to Improve Health Care Decision Making." *Health Services Research and Development Service.* www.hsrd.research.va.gov/publications/internal/outcomes.pdf.

# CHAPTER 6

# Costs and Cost-Finding in the Practice

## 6.1. Chapter Objectives

After completing the chapter you should be able to:

1. Define the main characteristics of cost behavior in ambulatory care practices.
2. Discuss the two types of cost analysis.
3. Compare and contrast four types of costing systems currently useful to ambulatory care practices.
4. Describe the organizational and policy uses of cost data.

## 6.2. Cost Behavior in Ambulatory Care Practices

Previously we discussed the need for health provider organizations to understand and respond to market incentives in order to succeed as a business. The reimbursement analysis outlined in Chapter 5 enables the practice to understand the market incentives that require a strategic response. The organization's financial plan that begins with a thorough reimbursement analysis (i.e., analysis of sources and methods of reimbursement) focuses on long- and short-term strategies to assure that there are payers for the provided healthcare and provider strategies match purchaser expectations. Costing is the next essential part of the organization's financial planning. Its purpose is to ensure that the provider's expenses are sufficient to meet care quality standards, do not exceed what purchasers are willing to pay, and enable net revenue (excess of revenue over costs) to expand the practice, reward investors, or provide a financial cushion for future upgrades or expansion. Understanding and controlling practice costs is necessary to price services and to plan and allocate practice revenue.

Practice costs have several important characteristics that need to be considered in financial planning. Table 6.1 illustrates the main types of costs and their characteristics.

Practice costs are defined by the commitment that is made when costs are incurred, the typical minimum time that can elapse before outlay is required, the duration of cost obligation, and the point at which costs can be terminated. Practice expenses may be classified into the traditional cost categories of property (real estate), labor, equipment, and supplies; however a small practice must understand in detail the nature of the commitment made when costs are incurred since this obligates funds that the practice cannot use for expansion, investment, or partner incentives. Cost duration and termination also defines the amount of financial "cushion" the practice should retain to assure orderly exit from the market if this becomes necessary.

Cost accountants typically classify costs in several ways. The classification of costs into *fixed*, *semi-variable*, and *fully variable* describes

TABLE 6.1. Main Characteristics of Practice Costs.

| Cost Category | Contract Vehicle | Typical Minimum Outlay Horizon | Cost Duration and Termination |
|---|---|---|---|
| Practice partner labor | Partnership agreement | Monthly | Contract terms |
| Fixed employee labor costs | Annual salary contract | Monthly | Two-weeks to one-month notice |
| Variable employee labor costs | Contractual | As specified in contract | Contract terms |
| Practice space | Rent contract or mortgage contract | Monthly or as specified in contract | Terms of lease, Terms of mortgage |
| Purchased patient care technology | Purchase terms | Monthly payment | Repayment cycle |
| Leased patient care technology | Lease terms | Monthly payment | Terms of lease |
| Fixed practice assets such as furniture and office equipment | Purchase terms | Monthly payment | Repayment cycle |
| Supplies | Invoice terms | Invoice terms upon receipt of invoice | Payment in full of invoice against payment terms |
| Utilities | Contract terms | Monthly payment | Terms of contract |

cost behavior in relation to volume. Fixed costs are those that do not vary with the volume of services provided. A typical example of such a cost is the payment for the physical space where the practice is located. This payment is typically made regardless of the number of patients or volume of care the practice provides. This is particularly true if the practice is purchasing the physical space, but even leased premises are fixed over a mid- to long-term horizon. Semi-variable costs are those in which a percentage of the cost varies with volume. Utilities are a good example of this type of cost. Some utility costs respond to clinical volume, e.g., electricity consumed by medical equipment; others do not, e.g., the telephone bill. Fully variable costs, such as disposable supplies used during a patient visit, change in direct proportion to the volume of patient visits. The horizon over which costs are fixed is an important consideration for a small practice because average annual costs are the usual basis for reimbursements to healthcare providers, and average cost can vary depending on market conditions. If provider revenue declines due to reduction in reimbursement rates, the practice needs to understand how soon it should increase the cost-efficiency of its operations in order to compensate for the impending shortfall of revenue. The key to this decision is the duration of contractual practice commitments (staff contracts, supplier contracts, space lease), an important feature in understanding the duration of fixed costs.

Cost traceability is another essential costing consideration. Cost accounting defines cost traceability in terms of direct costs, which can be traced directly to the services provided, and indirect costs, which cannot be directly linked to services. Tracing costs to services provided allows the practice to estimate the minimally acceptable reimbursement rates, observe cross-subsidization patterns, conduct break-even analysis, and address many other management needs with accurate cost information.

## 6.3.　Step-down Cost Analysis

Accurate cost tracking is key to effective financial management for at least two reasons: firstly, to help the practice set the charge for their services for reimbursement by the payers; secondly, to keep track of the costs of unreimbursed care in order to reflect them as business loss for tax purposes. Accurate cost tracking entails a complete allocation of costs of non-revenue-producing cost centers (practice units that do not bill the payer) to cost centers that do provide billable patient care and as such are termed revenue-producing cost centers. The task thus is to load patient care costs with practice overheads in a way that the payer will accept as reasonable and accurate.

This task is commonly solved by means of step-down cost allocation.

Medicare and many other purchasers of health care expect the use of this methodology by participating providers. The step-down cost allocation process comprises the following analytical and computational steps:

1. Identifying revenue-producing cost centers, i.e., organizational units that provide patient care and other billable services. Let us assume that the practice in case has Outpatient Clinics and Outpatient Surgery Center as the revenue-producing cost centers.

2. Identifying non-revenue-producing cost centers, i.e., organizational units that support revenue-earning centers but do not independently bill the purchasers of care for their costs. Physical Plant Management, Information Technology, General Administration, and Clinical Laboratory are the four non-revenue-producing cost centers in the analyzed practice. Their costs are referred to as practice overheads.

3. Calculating the total costs of revenue-producing and non-revenue-producing cost centers, as the total of their direct and indirect costs. Direct costs reflect resources that are easily traceable to a particular cost center, such as the cost center's full-time staff, equipment, furniture, and supplies. Indirect costs are those that are not easily traceable to a cost center, e.g., electricity, telephone, transport.

4. Establishing allocation criteria (otherwise referred to as cost drivers) to allocate the costs of non-revenue-producing cost centers to each other and to revenue-producing cost centers. For this purpose, the main function and associated cost should be determined for each non-revenue-producing cost center. The Physical Plant Management spends its budget primarily in lease payments on behalf of the practice. A reasonable assumption is that lease should be spread across the other cost centers proportionately to their floor space. In addition to lease, Physical Plant Management incurs such costs as repair and maintenance. However, since lease payments are identified as the main cost, the cost driver chosen for the lease (i.e., floor space) will apply to this cost center's total cost. Similarly, the costs of IT will be spread across the other cost centers proportionately to the number of work stations in each unit. The cost driver for General Administration can be defined as the direct cost of each patient care unit. The underlying assumption is that a costlier unit would require more support from practice administration. Finally, the cost driver for Clinical Laboratory would be an RVU-adjusted[1] number of tests ordered by each patient care unit.

---

[1]RVUs are relative value units: cost weights assigned to each service. Services that involve more resources and therefore are costlier will be characterized by higher RVUs. The 'average service' has RVU = 1. See more in the next section.

5. Allocating the costs of non-revenue-producing cost centers to the other cost centers, using the allocation statistics selected in Step 4.
6. Summing up the direct and indirect costs by revenue-producing unit to estimate the total cost of patient care.

Table 6.2 illustrates the step-down allocation process as described in steps 1 to 6. The term 'step-down', by the way, is invoked by the staircase-shaped cluster of numbers in the right part of the table.

Let us take a close look at the computations in Table 6.2:

- Column F is the sum of Columns D and E.
- The shaded cells K1, L2, M3 and N4 feature the total costs of non-revenue-producing units as a respective unit's cost (Column F) plus a fraction of costs allocated from other non-revenue-producing cost centers. Thus Cell K1 = F1. Cell L2 = F2 + K2. Cell M3 = F3 + K3 + L3. Cell N4 = F4 + Sum(K4:M4).
- Cell K2 = K1 * G2 / G7 = $450,000 * 250(sq.ft) / 9,550(sq.ft) = $11,780. In words, Information Technology assumes the percentage of costs of 'Physical Plant Management' that equals the IT's percent share in the practice's total floor space.
- Column O = Columns K + L + M + N.
- Column P = Columns F + O.
- Numbers in Cells F7 and P7 are the same: the practice's total cost initially aggregated from direct costs of all the cost centers (cell F7) has been 'compressed' to the total cost of revenue-earning units (cells P5 and P6) as the result of step-down cost allocation.

A few concluding insights into the reviewed cost allocation algorithm:

1. The costs of non-revenue-producing units are allocated in the 'downward' manner: to those units that are lower on the cost center list (Column B, Table 6.2) but not to those that are above. Thus, Information Technology is treated as a consumer of services of Physical Plant Management but not the other way around. This is not true to life but is an acceptable simplification, since ultimately the costs of both units are passed down to revenue-producing cost centers.
2. Sometimes, the step-down cost allocation process is set up to apportion the costs of non-revenue-producing units to revenue-producing units only. The cost flows shown in Table 6.2 reflect a

TABLE 6.2. Step-down Cost Allocation: An Illustrative Case of an Outpatient Practice.

| | | Cost by Cost Center | | | Cost drivers: statistics for allocation of costs of non-revenue-producing units | | | | Step-down allocation of total costs of non-revenue-producing cost centers | | | | | |
|---|---|---|---|---|---|---|---|---|---|---|---|---|---|---|
| | Organizational Units (Cost Centers) | Direct costs | Indirect costs | Total costs before step-down | Floor space, sq.ft | Work stations | Direct costsl | RVU-adjusted tests | Physical Plant | IT | Gen Admin | Lab | Sub-total: Over-heads | TOTAL COSTS after step-down allocation |
| B | C | D | E | F | G | H | I | J | K | L | M | N | O | P |
| 1 | Physical Plant Management | $ 300,000 | 120,000 | $ 420,000 | | | | | $ 420,000 | | | | | |
| 2 | Information Technology | $ 80,000 | 70,000 | $ 150,000 | 250 | | | | $ 10,959 | $160,995 | | | | |
| 3 | General Administration | $ 120,000 | 30,000 | $ 150,000 | 300 | 10 | | | $ 13,194 | $ 33,541 | $196,734 | | | |
| 4 | Clinical Laboratory | $ 200,000 | 150,000 | $ 350,000 | 5,000 | 8 | $ 350,000 | | $219.895 | $ 26,832 | $ 20,554 | $617,282 | | |
| 5 | Outpatient Clinics | $1,000,000 | 300,000 | $ 1,300,000 | 3,000 | 25 | $1,300,000 | 45,000 | $ 131,937 | $ 83,851 | $ 76,345 | $555,554 | $ 847,687 | $ 2,147,687 |
| 6 | Outpatient Surgery | $ 800,000 | 900,000 | $ 1,700,000 | 1,000 | 5 | $1,700.000 | 5,000 | $ 43,979 | $ 16,700 | $ 99,835 | $ 61.728 | $ 222,313 | $ 1,922,313 |
| 7 | Total | $2,500,000 | $ 1,570,000 | $ 4,070,000 | 9,550 | 48 | $3,350,000 | 50,000 | | | | | $1,070,000 | $ 4,070,000 |

Rows 1–4: Non-revenue producing
Rows 5–6: Revenue producing

74

more nuanced approach whereby the non-revenue-producing units allocate costs both to each other and the revenue-producing units.

3. The distinction between producers and non-producers of revenue is fluid. If Clinical Laboratory starts serving externally referred patients, it will bill the referring providers for part of its services. Thus, it will become a partially revenue-producing cost center. The numbers on line 4 and particularly the Lab's total cost in cell 'N4' (Table 6.2) will inform the pricing of clinical lab tests for direct billing.

4. The step-down cost analysis is not a rigid approach but rather an algorithm that flexibly responds to the cost analysis needs of practice management and providers of care. The next section gives additional insight into the analytic agenda and cost assessment tools of a healthcare practice.

## 6.4.  Costing Systems Useful to Ambulatory Care Practices

The previous discussion of direct and indirect cost analysis provides an insight into the importance of systematic approaches to cost analysis. However costs need to be analyzed in a context. For example, it is difficult to determine if costs are excessive unless the practice also considers productivity, the ratio of revenue to costs, and the outcomes of care. Selection of the appropriate contextual analytics used to understand practice costs should always be done with consideration of the payer base, the complexity of the practice, and the cost of implementing the analytical system.

Relative value units (RVUs) are assigned by Medicare and can be used to compare practice cost and productivity with a regional and national standard. A practice that intends to accept Medicare payment should develop a clear understanding of RVUs, which are the productivity measures on which Medicare reimbursement is based. Each service-specific RVU is a ratio that relates the cost of a service to the average cost across all the services. RVUs are developed by analyzing three factors: (1) average practice expense, which reflects both the direct and indirect costs of providing services, (2) malpractice expense, and (3) physician-provider work, which includes an empirically based estimate of the provider's time, skill, judgment, and training required for a given service. RVUs are national average values derived from data obtained from the American Medical Association's Physician Practice Information Survey. RVUs are revised annually and published by Centers for Medicare and Medicaid Services in the *Federal Register*, first in preliminary form for comment and then final form three to six months later.

In order to determine the payment that can be expected based on the RVUs delivered, the practice must also consider the Geographic Practice Cost Index (GPCI), which is used in conjunction with the RVU to adjust the payment, depending on the location of the practice. The GPCI is applied to each component of the RVU calculation in order to determine the full RVU weight that is assigned to a specific service. The standard formula for calculating the service-specific RVU is:

$$\text{Practice expense RVU} \times \text{Practice Expense GPCI} + \text{Malpractice RVU} \times \text{Malpractice GPCI} + \text{Physician work RVU} \times \text{Physician Work GPCI} = \text{Total RVU}$$

The service-specific payment amount equals the current Medicare Conversion Factor (CF) multiplied by Total RVU. The conversion factor is a dollar amount proposed annually by CMS and approved by Congress.

Practices can examine productivity by analyzing the number of RVUs delivered by the practice as a whole or by each provider in the practice. The practice can also compute its average cost per RVU by dividing practice costs by the number of RVUs delivered over a defined period of time. Understanding RVU delivery and cost structure in a given practice provides an important context for cost analysis. This is particularly important since Medicare payment is based on a set conversion of RVUs to dollar amounts derived from the sector-wide costs and regardless of practice-specific costs. A practice with costs per RVU in excess of the reimbursable level will quickly have to find alternative revenue sources or go out of business. For practices with a large Medicare patient base, careful monitoring of the cost per RVU is essential.

The ratio of costs to charges (RCC) is also a useful contextual tool that provides information on the revenue capacity of the practice. This method is particularly useful when detailed cost data are not available but cost estimates are needed quickly, for example, to evaluate potential contracts. A cost to charge ratio is compiled by taking the total costs of a practice over a defined period and dividing them by the total amount billed during the same period. This ratio is then used to project costs from anticipated contract revenue as long as the contract is not expected to include patients that are markedly different than those already served by the practice. Since many payers stipulate a payment schedule that does not consider practice costs, the RCC provides a way for the practice to decide whether to accept the proposed contract. Primary care practices that have a limited scope of services are particularly well positioned to use the RCC tool to estimate the anticipated costs of a given contract because the variation in services delivered by the practice is small. Research suggests that determination of the cost of an individual patient using the RCC method is not reliable. Aggregate analysis of expected costs of a group is much more stable (Swartz, Young, and Siegrist 1995). The RCC should not substitute for a detailed analysis of the practice costs, but it can expedite decision making when detailed data is not available, as is the case with a new contract.

The activity-based costing (ABC) as a direct-costing approach is part of a cost-analysis system developed to support more precise management decision-making relevant to cost control in manufacturing (Fritzch 1998). As manufacturing competition increased, it became important to understand cost drivers with more specificity. ABC begins with the product or service as the basic analytic unit. The analysis is built by tracing all costs to the service produced. For example, an ABC cost analysis measures the amount of supervisory time actually delivered rather than using a formula based on the number of employees in the unit that delivered the service. It is easy to see that ABC costing systems increase the precision of cost analysis. Managers can compare services based on the actual total cost required to produce these services. They can also understand where costs can be reduced without compromising service quality. For example, if the analysis shows that a primary care visit is absorbing an excessive amount of the management overhead in a practice, methods for reducing the dependence of the primary care team on management can be designed. Improved employee training, increased experience or training requirements for staff, or better information support can decrease administrative overhead. In this example the number of staff who deliver the service might not change, but the quality and knowledge support given to the staff would improve. Step-down cost allocation would not provide the detailed evidence needed to support this type of management decision or evaluate changes made in management structure, but ABC costing would.

The amount of information required to implement an ABC analysis is considerable. Cost tracing must be detailed and precise. There also must be ongoing costing systems in place to monitor cost behavior at the service level to support and evaluate management decision making. However, the information gained with the ABC costing method is considerable, and it enables management to address organizational costs with precision. In the highly regulated healthcare delivery environment, the investment in the ABC approach, particularly in a very competitive market, can help ensure practice survival.

The implementation of accountable care organizations (ACO) introduces a need for costing systems that can evaluate costs across organizational boundaries. The ACO is an approach designed by Medicare to support better cost control without a decrease in quality of care. The ACO consists of a network of providers that earn additional revenue if they can provide the same or better quality in an episode of care at a lower than average cost. The unit of analysis in the ACO is a defined episode of care tied to a diagnostic group comprised of many related services delivered to a Medicare beneficiary. One episode of care might be focused on total hip replacement. This care episode might consist of outpatient and inpatient surgical care as well as skilled nursing care and physical therapy. The total cost of the care episode is considered regardless of the organizational boundaries that previously existed for the care team. To provide care for the entire defined episode, a new umbrella organization is formed specifically to carefully manage service delivery and costs across the entire continuum of care for the enrolled patient. The ACO is a separate legal entity formed for this purpose by one or more Medicare-enrolled healthcare providers or suppliers (Internal Revenue Service, 2011). These providers may continue to see other non-ACO patients, but for those that are in the ACO the normal organizational boundaries do not apply. Specific ACO costing systems have yet to be fully defined. However, it is clear that ACOs will depend heavily on shared data systems that have common cost definitions, can trace costs directly to services provided, and can provide detailed and compatible service costing reports. The use of direct cost tracing for the ACO portion of a provider's patient base will become increasingly necessary as ACO organizations assume financial risk since management of this risk depends directly on understanding the costs involved for each ACO provider. Practices considering ACO participation should develop a clear understanding of the information system requirements as well as the additional cost information that will be required to evaluate financial risk against return. Current information suggests that direct-costing systems such as ABC will be necessary to assure financial survival in the ACO market (Turcan, 2012).

### 6.5.  The Organizational and Policy Uses of Cost Data

Practice organizations engage cost data to understand financial resource use in the context of the total practice or at the level of individual service providers within the practice. When the practice is the target of cost analysis, the questions typically focus on the contribution of cost to practice financial performance. Break-even analysis is a common financial tool that is used to look at practice costs in the context. The question posed by break-even analysis is a seemingly simple one: At what operational point has a practice earned enough revenue to recoup its costs? Inherent in this question is the understanding that some portions of the operations represent variable costs that are incurred by each unit of service. These costs are incurred each time a service is delivered.

$$[(\text{Work RVU} \times \text{Work GPCI}) + (\text{PER VU} \times \text{RE GPCI}) + (\text{MP RVU} \times \text{MP GPCI})] \times \text{CF}$$

**FIGURE 6.1.** *Medicare Professional Fee Schedule (PFS) payment rates formula.*

Fixed costs, on the other hand, are incurred when the practice begins and must be paid regardless of the operational volume. If a practice delivers just enough services to pay the fixed plus the variable costs of its service volume, then it is said to break even. At this point the practice receives enough revenue to meet its financial obligations, but it makes no additional profit. Below the break-even point the practice cannot meet its costs. The level above break-even that the practice chooses to operate is a strategic decision based on the revenue expectations of the practice partners and an understanding of the market in which the practice operates. As the break-even analysis illustrates, an understanding of the practice cost behavior is the first step in defining the financial and investment strategy of the practice. This is particularly true in a market where the ability to increase service charges is limited by provider competition, government policy and a growing role of payers who favor charge-based or discounted charge-based payments. In such markets, control of practice costs is the main strategy to ensure a sufficient level of revenue to continue operations, a level of return on investment in the practice, and adequate investments in practice technology.

Practice cost data is used for payment decisions that affect the delivery of ambulatory care not only to Medicare and Medicaid patients but also to private insurers who tend to mirror policy reimbursement decisions made by the public sector payers.

Figure 6.1 presents the Medicare Professional Fee Schedule (PFS) payment rates formula as described in the Medicare Claims Processing Manual (Centers for Medicare and Medicaid Services, 2012). This fee schedule consists of four main elements that are adjusted by the geographic practice cost indices (GPCI), which set the national relative value unit by geographic variation in each element:

1. Work = the physician work unit, which is the amount of time it takes a physician to provide a particular service.
2. PE = the expenses required to provide services in the office. These expenses are the typical cost drivers discussed in this chapter. These include rent or lease payments, labor costs, supply costs, and other direct and indirect costs necessary to provide services.
3. MP = malpractice costs, which are the costs of malpractice insurance for providers in the practice.

4. CF = a conversion factor that is recommended annually by CMS to Congress. It is defined by statute to include analysis of four factors: the increase in provider fees paid by the private sector, the increase in Medicare enrollment, the increase in the ten-year moving average gross domestic product, and any increase or decrease due to changes in law or regulation.

The most direct reflection of practice cost data is in the practice expense index, which is estimated annually. Currently the practice expense data is based on the American Medical Association's Physician Practice Information Survey data, which reflect practice expenses of physicians and non-physician practitioners (Centers for Medicare and Medicaid Services, 2013). The nonphysician practitioners included in the 2008 survey were audiologists, chiropractors, clinical psychologists, clinical social workers, optometrists, oral surgeons, physical therapists, podiatrists, and registered dieticians (American Medical Association, 2009). Practice costs are also indirectly considered in the annual conversion fee calculation because provider fees paid by the private sector are based, in part, on the cost of providing care.

The PFS has a profound influence on provider reimbursement both by public and private payers. Some commercial payers directly link to the PFS, some apply a percentage adjustment to the PFS payment, and some apply a different geographic conversion adjustment or a different conversion factor (Baker and Baker, 2011). Therefore it is in the best interests of any ambulatory care provider to have a clear and precise understanding of not only their own cost structure, but also the average costs of providers of ambulatory care in their geographic area as well as nationally.

The tools and methods discussed in this chapter are intended as a basis for further discussion with financial and accounting professionals as well as to provide basic information to the practitioner intending to manage practice costs. In summary, cost management is one of the most important financial aspects of healthcare delivery and should be the concern of all health professionals involved in ambulatory care.

## 6.6.  Concept Checkout

Be sure you understand these concepts before you begin the discussion questions:

- Fixed, semi-variable, and variable costs
- Direct and indirect costs
- Step-down cost allocation

- Relative value units
- Ratio of costs to charges
- Activity-based costing
- Accountable care organizations
- Public and private uses of cost data

## 6.7. Discussion Questions

1. Review the list of practice expenses provided (see page 70) and classify each as fixed, semi-variable, or variable. Give a brief rationale for your classification decision.
2. You have been asked to conduct a cost-finding analysis for your practice. One of the first activities you undertake is the classification of costs into direct and indirect categories. Explain how you will classify the costs and give a rationale from the literature to support your classification method.
3. Define and give an example of step-down cost allocation as part of your definition. Discuss the strengths and challenges in activity-based costing or step-down cost allocation.
4. Select one of the costing systems reviewed in this chapter and discuss in detail how this system could be applied to an ambulatory practice. Your discussion should consider (1) the data required to analyze practice costs using the system, (2) the analytical approach to use, and (3) the major advantages of using the system you have chosen.
5. You have been asked to participate in the Physician Practice Information Survey. The other partners in your practice do not understand why the practice should take the time to participate. Give a brief rationale (not more than two pages) that supports participation in this survey.

## 6.8. References

American Medical Association. 2007. Physician Practice Information Survey Overview. American Medical Association.

Baker, J., and R. W. Baker. 2011. Health Care Finance: Basic Tools for Nonfinancial Managers. Burlington, Mass.: Jones and Bartlett Learning.

Centers for Medicare and Medicaid. 2012. Medicare Claims Processing Manual, Rev 2464. www.cms.gov/Medicare/Medicare-Fee-for-Service-Payment/PhysicianFee-Sched/index.html?redirect=/physicianfeesched/.

———. 2013. Medicare Physician Fee Schedule Fact Sheet. www.cms.gov/Outreach-and-Education/Medicare-Learning-Network-MLN/MLNProducts/downloads/Med-crePhysFeeSchedfctsht.pdf.

Fritzch, R. 1998. "Activity-Based Costing and the Theory of Constraints." *Journal of Applied Business Research* 14 (1): 83–89.

Internal Revenue Service. 2011. "Tax-Exempt Organizations Participating in the Medicare Shared Savings Program through Accountable Care Organizations." Fact Sheet FS-2011-11. www.irs.gov/uac/Tax-Exempt-Organizations-Participating-in-the-Medicare-Shared-Savings-Program-through-Accountable-Care-Organizations.

Swartz , M., D. Young, and R. Siegrist. 1995. "The Ratio of Costs to Charges: How Good a Basis for Estimating Costs?" *Inquiry* 32:476–81.

Turcan, D. 2012a. "Must-Have ACO Infrastructure." Executive Insight column posted August 17, 2012. *Advance Healthcare Network.* http://healthcare-executive-insight.advanceweb.com/Columns/ACO-Acumen/Must-Have-ACO-Infrastructure.aspx

———. 2012b. "Must-Have Infrastructure for Accountable Care Organizations." Posted December 28, 2012. *Advance Healthcare Network.* http://health-information.advanceweb.com/Features/Articles/Must-Have-Infrastructure-for-Accountable-Care-Organizations.aspx.

# Homegrown Healthcare Inc.: A Rural Accountable Care Organization

*You should not attempt this case until you have completed Chapters 1–6 of the textbook.*

*The facts in the case:*

Homegrown Healthcare operates in a nonmetropolitan county that contains an urban population of 2,500–19,999, with one small city and an adjacent urban county containing a larger metropolitan center. Homegrown Healthcare has its offices in the small city located in the northeast corner of the county. The demographics of the county are as shown in Table CS3.1.

The county has a 55-bed nonprofit acute care hospital with an average occupancy rate of 90 percent.

**Ambulatory Medicine**

There are five primary care practice groups and one independent internal medicine physician with a specialization in preventive medicine. There are specialty practices in ophthalmology, orthopedics, surgery, podiatry, radiology, and pediatrics. All primary care practices and the internal medicine physician accept Medicare.

There are three small intermediate care facilities in the county for the elderly and others requiring intermediate care. The hospital has a subacute unit that is qualified as a skilled nursing facility.

Homegrown is one of the five primary care group practices in the county. It is located near the rural hospital, and the hospital has approached Homegrown, the orthopedic practice, and the surgical practice

*TABLE CS3.1. County Demographics.*

| | |
|---|---|
| Population (2010 Census) | 30,097 |
| Population Distribution (known ages only) | |
|     Under 5 | 1,520 (5.1%) |
|     5–19 | 5,591 (18.9%) |
|     20–44 | 8,757 (29.6%) |
|     45–64 | 8,546 (28.9%) |
|     65 + | 5,141 (17.4%) |
|     **Total** | **29,555** |
| Median Age | 42.2 years |
| Employment (Total Civilian Labor Force) | |
|     Employed | 15,138 |
|     Unemployed | 1,354 |
| Residents Commuting Outside the County to Work | 3,066  (21.4%) |
| Employment in Selected Occupations | |
|     Management/Professional | 29.4% of employed workers |
|     Service | 18.1% |
|     Sales and Office | 20.1% |
|     Production, Transportation, and Material Moving | 15.5% |
| Educational Attainment | |
|     High School Graduates or higher | 84.8% |
|     Bachelor's Degree or higher | 17.7% |

*TABLE CS3.2. Major Health Indicators.*

| | |
|---|---|
| Life Expectancy at Birth | 77.9 |
| % With Activity Limitations | 22.5 |
| % With Fair or Poor Health | 14.8 |
| % Experiencing Unhealthy Days | 18.4 |
| All-cause Mortality  (100,000 population) | 789.1 |
| Infant Mortality Rate | NA |
| % Low Birth Weight (Singleton) | 4.7 |
| % Low Birth Weight (All) | 6.5 |
| % Very Low Birth Weight (Singleton) | NA |
| % Very Low Birth Weight (All) | NA |
| % Pre-Term Births | 7.6 |
| Teen Birth Rate | NA |
| Tuberculosis Incidence  (per 100,000) | 3.4 |
| Chlamydia Incidence (per 100,000) | 50.9 |
| Gonorrhea Incidence  (per 100,000) | 10.2 |
| Incidence of HIV/AIDS Cases  (per 100,000) | 0.0 |
| Number of HIV Deaths | 1 |
| Number of Septicemia Deaths | 3 |

TABLE CS3.3. Health Outcomes/Risk Factors.

| | |
|---|---|
| Number of Suicide Deaths | 0 |
| % with Anxiety Disorders | 10.7 |
| Number of Alcohol-Induced Deaths | 3 |
| % Binge Drinkers | 11.3 |
| % Children Tested for Presence of Blood Lead | 19.4 |
| % Children With Lead Poisoning | 0.4 |
| % Without Health Insurance (Adults) | NA |
| % Without Health Insurance (Children) | NA |
| % in Last Year that Could Not Afford to See a Doctor | 12.7 |
| % That did not see a Dentist in the Last Year | 28.6 |

to form an ACO. The initial meeting among the partners was lengthy. The hospital requested all partners to review the literature on ACOs and become familiar with CMS's general structure and plan for participating organizations. All participants were referred to the Medicare Learning Network on the CMS website for helpful background information.

The application to form a new ACO was then presented to meeting participants and every participant was requested to select one of the clinical focus areas in and draft a response to the focus area questions.

You are Homegrown's expert in healthcare finance and you were asked to focus on the following question which speaks to cost and quality metrics:

### Internally Reporting on Quality and Cost Metrics

37. Submit a narrative describing how the ACO defines, establishes, implements, evaluates, and periodically updates its process and infrastructure to support internal reporting on quality and cost metrics that lets the ACO monitor, give feedback, and evaluate ACO participant and ACO provider/supplier perfomance. Also, describe how you use these results to improve care and service over time. Also describe how the ACO will use the internal assessments of this process to continuously improve the ACO's care practices.

*From: Centers for Medicare and Medicaid Services. Medicare Shared Savings Program Application. 2013.*

Your task is to discuss the data you need to analyze the cost savings that result from coordination of care and increased quality that the ACO will deliver. You decide to focus on one area of practice as an example and select total hip replacement as the focus because this condition requires input from all partners in the ACO. Please remember that the hospital has a subacute unit that is qualified to deliver skilled nursing care eligible for Medicare reimbursement for rehabilitation therapy.

TABLE CS3.4. Chronic Disease Trends and Screening Rates.

| | |
|---|---|
| Number of Colorectal Cancer Deaths | 10 |
| Number of Breast Cancer Deaths | 7 |
| Number of Heart Disease Deaths | 75 |
| Number of Stroke Deaths | 21 |
| % with Diabetes | 10.0 |
| Diabetes Deaths** | NA |
| % Children with Asthma | 10.0 |
| Number of Childhood Asthma Hospitalizations | 6 |
| % Adults with Asthma | 10.7 |
| Number of Adult Asthma Hospitalizations | 24 |
| % Adult Women that have Received a Mammogram | 62.5 |
| % Screened for Colorectal Cancer in Last 2 Years | 18.6 |

Your analysis should consider the following questions:

1. What general financial-data categories are necessary to estimate the costs involved in the total hip replacement across all the levels of care, and what concerns do you have about cost reporting across all participating organizations?
2. Discuss at least three major considerations that you will define to ensure accuracy in cost reporting.
3. Outline at least one method of cost reporting that you will suggest to ensure that all organizations actively manage their patient-care costs and take corrective action quickly if costs exceed reasonable limits.
4. Outline a cost-accounting SWOT analysis focused on the costing system needs of the new ACO. You will need to research the current risks and benefits contained in the ACO approach as well as the particular risks of rural ACOs.

TABLE CS3.5. Immunization Rates and Environmental Determinants.

| | |
|---|---|
| Average % of Kindergarten Students Immunized | 100.0 |
| % Adults Receiving Flu Shots | 36.7 |
| % Adults Receiving Pneumonia Shots | 23.5 |
| Ozone Days | 1 |
| Particulate Matter Days | 0 |
| Water Quality—Arsenic † | 10.9 |
| Water Quality—Nitrates ‡ | NA |
| Water Quality—Trihalomethane † | NA |
| Water Quality—Haloecetic Acids † | NA |

5. Discuss the role of shared strategic planning and expense budgeting in managing ACO performance in providing a hip-replacement episode of care. Remember that the goal of the ACO is to demonstrate cost savings over the current fragmented method of delivering hip-replacement surgery.

Please assume that the new ACO will elect to participate in the track 1 option that calculates shared savings only for the first performance year. The ACO will not assume any financial risk during this first year. Remember, however, that after the first year all ACOs will have to assume financial risk. You may make any other reasonable assumption necessary to discuss the case. Do not, however, assume that all nascent ACO partners have compatible EMR and accounting systems, because this is highly unlikely. You may assume that all potential ACO partners are currently on a sound financial footing, that none are at risk of bankruptcy, and all have the necessary practice and administration staff to develop essential ACO systems.

# Section 4

# CHAPTER 7

# Revenue Planning and Management

## 7.1. Chapter Objectives

After completing the chapter you should be able to:

1. Discuss the main points to be considered in a revenue management plan.
2. Explain the strategies necessary for revenue account management.
3. Define revenue optimization objectives and revenue account evaluation.
4. Outline the strategies for revenue account negotiation based on practice revenue requirements.

## 7.2. Managing Revenue

In Chapter 5 we discussed the need for a reimbursement plan that outlines the beneficiary base, the services that are reimbursed, how reimbursement is requested and received, the payer's incentive and penalty structure, and who within the practice may bill. The reimbursement plan is an essential part of the information the practice needs for each prospective payer. The information collected in the reimbursement plan is used to define an operational revenue plan and budget. The operations side of revenue planning is focused on the details of billing, payment receipts, evaluation of payment sources, and renegotiation of payer contracts based on payment considerations.

## Managing the Payment-to-Provider Process

Revenue receipt depends on complete and accurate billing. The practice manager must see to it that the bills contain all the information required by the payer. These requirements typically establish *who* can submit a bill, *what* format the bill must follow, *what* services can be billed, *when* the bill can be submitted, *when* payment can be expected, and *where* the bill should be sent. Proper management of accounts receivable depends on this information since almost no healthcare services are delivered on a cash basis. When a practice bills for services, it is extending credit to the payer because services are provided before payment is received. Extension of credit is a form of loan, and the provider critically depends on prompt payment to remain a viable business. It is easy to understand this point if you consider the typical flow of funds from a practice on a monthly basis. A practice usually must pay for rent, utilities, salaries, and supplies on a 30-day cycle. If payers reimburse on a 90- to 120-day cycle, the provider must have enough cash on hand to pay for three to four months of expenses before sufficient funds are received to cover the first month's costs. This revenue cycle suggests that the provider can expect to finance at least three months of expenses on a permanent basis because the revenue received will always lag expenditures at this time interval.

If the practice does not have sufficient cash to cover at least three months of expenditures, a short-term loan or line of credit will have to be negotiated to continue service delivery. This need for short-term credit means that the practice faces the need to expend some funds on interest payments. Because short-term interest rates are usually higher than long-term rates, this cost may be significant. The longer this interval becomes, the more interest the practice pays. Because payers usually do not pay for finance charges, the practice must reduce revenue by the amount it costs to provide funds for this period or include the requisite amount in the overhead rate that it charges the payer, if the payer will accept overhead charges. If the payer does not accept overhead charges, then the practice must include this cost as a charge against revenues received. This is why slow payers may be said to significantly increase the real cost of healthcare delivery.

To minimize overhead costs, the provider needs to consider the interval between billing and revenue receipt when negotiating payment terms with suppliers. Many suppliers do not accept payment cycles longer than 30 days from delivery, but some suppliers will negotiate the length of the payment cycle. Providers who clearly understand the conditions for payment defined in their payer contracts are in a favorable position to negotiate better payment terms from their suppliers.

Many financial operations planners suggest matching accounts payable and receivable so that the interval for payment of suppliers and receipt of revenue is the same. In healthcare this is difficult to arrange because the major costs of a practice are in salaries and technology acquired by lease or loan financing that must be paid monthly. However, wherever possible it is wise to negotiate a longer payment cycle with suppliers, lessors, and lenders that more closely matches the payment receipt cycle.

## Managing Revenue Receipts in the Practice

When payment is received for services, careful attention should be paid to matching the payment to the invoice or bill. For most patient care services there are two kinds of payment: the co-payment that the patient makes and the payment that the insurer makes. The co-payment is usually collected at the time of service while the insurer's payment is made after the bill is submitted in the proper format to the insurer. It is important to collect the correct information from the patient at the time of service so that insurers are billed properly and co-payments or deductibles are correctly accounted. In the case of Medicare, new patients should always complete the Medicare secondary-payer questionnaire so that the practice can determine the primary payer for a medical claim and submit the initial invoice to the correct payer. The Medicare fact sheet on secondary payment is a helpful first step to understand primary and secondary payment for Medicare beneficiaries (Centers for Medicare and Medicaid Services, 2012).

In order to strengthen the accounts-receivable process, the practice is advised to complete reimbursement analysis on each payer it plans to invoice. The correct primary payer should be determined for each patient, and the bill should be submitted in the proper format to the correctly identified payment source. After co-payments, deductible payments, and primary payments are collected, the total revenue received for the service should equal the revenue expected unless claims were denied or excluded. At this point, matching the revenue received with the revenue expected is important. If a balance remains, practice administrators must decide if a secondary payer can be billed for the uncollected portion of the account or if the patient can be billed. Before billing either a secondary payer or the patient, the reimbursement agreements with the primary payer should be carefully reviewed.

The amount billed must be in accordance with the agreed-on fee schedule. The portion of the claim that was not paid must fall within the defined limits of services that can be billed to the secondary payer or patient. Balance billing—billing for charges in excess of agreed-on fee schedules—is generally not allowed by major payers. Once a contract between a provider and a payer is agreed to, the provider cannot bill the patient or a secondary payer for fees in excess of fee schedule. Providers must also make a good-faith effort to collect co-payments and deductibles that are owed under the terms of agreements with insurers or public payers such as Medicare, Medicaid, or Workman's Compensation. These payments cannot usually be waived by the provider because to do so might constitute fraud. Occasional exceptions in the case of medically indigent patients may be allowed, but routine waiver of deductibles and co-payments violates the agreed-on billing policies and should be avoided. In general, billing practices should conform to the terms and conditions that were agreed to when the practice accepted the payer contract. The financial manager should ensure that accurate bills are issued in accordance with these terms and conditions and that all revenue expected is collected.

### 7.3. Allocating Revenue to Accounts: The Account Management Challenge

The management of revenue accounts greatly benefits from an accurate decomposition of the patient-payer-service mix, description of the services delivered to the patients, including correct coding, review of allowable billing and claims submission requirements, correct posting of payments received and payment denials, payment appeals analysis, and subsequent patient management at the individual and group level.

The practice should establish clear revenue-management policy with indicator monitoring that provides all practice managers with the information needed to detect problems in revenue accounts. Many firms offer revenue management services to providers. Selection of a firm to manage this important part of the practice should be done carefully and with some basic knowledge of adequate revenue cycle management. This section presents basic concepts that providers need in order to make informed decisions on revenue cycle management.

Revenue management can be divided into three phases that are informed by accounts-receivable performance indicators: pre-encounter administration, encounter management, and post-encounter revenue administration (TripleTree Industry Analysis, 2006).

The pre-encounter phase includes two main activities: eligibility determination and benefit authorization. When a prospective patient contacts the provider for an appointment, a decision-tree analysis should be activated to guide practice staff through a series of service questions that define the patient's eligibility. It is easy to see how important the reimbursement analysis phase is to this activity. Practice staff need to know if the prospective patient belongs to a group authorized to seek care from the provider as well as determining if the service likely to be requested is authorized and under what conditions. For example, if preauthorization is necessary for the requested service, it must be obtained before the provider encounter. If the practice has done a good job of reimbursement analysis for each payer group, these questions can be quickly answered from the reimbursement or payer database. The practice may choose from a variety of pre-encounter forms that collect information and link to practice reimbursement data. Regardless of the method of managing the pre-encounter phase, the following basic questions need to be answered to qualify the patient and correctly refer an ineligible patient to an alternative provider: (1) Is the patient a member of a group qualified to seek care from the provider? (2) Is the requested service authorized under the terms of the group agreement with the provider?

The second phase of revenue management is centered on the patient encounter, which begins when the patient arrives for the appointment. Basic activities in this phase are focused on the pre-service encounter, the provider service encounter, and the post-service encounter. The pre-service encounter should assure that all required co-payments are collected and that payment and claim information is accurate and current. Most practices have patients complete a pre-encounter form that collects this information. The pre-encounter form is completed and reviewed by practice staff, the insurance information is verified, the required copayment is collected, and any clinical information requested is checked and provided to the clinical staff. If an electronic medical record is available, the accuracy of registry information included in the record should be verified with the patient before the clinical encounter.

The post-service encounter begins when the patient and provider meet and ends when the provider delivers the clinical service and provides any required aftercare information to the patient. Reimbursement-related activities in this phase focus on correct description of the service, accurate data and coding entry, and documentation of any needed follow-up services. In the clinical encounter phase, providers need to be aware of all coding requirements, any referral restrictions or documentation requirements, and the conditions that must be met before diagnostic tests of prescriptions can be entered. Additionally, the clinician needs to consider the requirements for follow-up care, if this is indicated, or for referral to other clinical providers if necessary. During the encounter phase, quality-of-care considerations are also important. For example, many payers are now requiring significant health and illness prevention education to decrease unnecessary utilization and assure good understanding of aftercare requirements. It is important to be sure that these requirements are met and documented as part of the service encounter.

During the post-service encounter, the practice staff completes the billing of the encounter by editing and submitting the provider's bill for services. If the pre-encounter and encounter phases were correctly managed, the post-encounter billing should go smoothly without payment denials or other problems. Preparation of a "clean" bill that is promptly submitted for payment and paid within the payers' defined window is the goal. Appeals for nonpayment, bills returned due to improper coding, or disallowed services are indicators of problems in reimbursement analysis and revenue management. These delays in revenue collection represent a resource drain for the practice because revenue that is not received on time requires additional use of credit to pay expenses. As we have seen, credit adds to the increased cost of care for the practice and ultimately for society.

## 7.4.  Revenue Optimization and Account Evaluation

The two main indicators that should be routinely followed in revenue accounts are (1) time in accounts receivable (AR), and (2) aging analysis. These indicators, if computed for each payer on a routine basis, will signal areas of revenue collection that need additional attention.

---

How to compute days in accounts receivable (Days in AR):

1. Compute your total charges for a defined period of time.
2. Divide by the number of days in that time period. The result is the average daily charge.
3. Divide the total in your accounts receivable by the average daily charges. This is the average number of days it is taking you to collect your payments for bills submitted.

---

Here is an example: You charged $500,000 for services you delivered in the past six months. If there were 180 days in these months, then your average daily charges are $2,777.79. If your accounts receivables right now is $125,000, then the days in AR is 45 (125,000/2777.79). This means it is taking 45 days to receive payment against the account.

Benchmarking services can provide you with national and regional norms against which to judge your AR performance. Or you can trend your performance and take action when your days in AR exceed payment terms and conditions from your suppliers. Your account evaluation should include the days in AR for each payer account as well as evaluation of billing problems such as denied claims, coding or claims errors, and successful and unsuccessful appeals.

Payer experience is a fundamental part of your practice management strategy, and payer problems should be managed by terminating problem-fraught contracts or negotiating with payers for better claims-management protocols.

## 7.5. Account Negotiation Strategies

Negotiations with payers should be evidence-based. Data from initial reimbursement analysis as well as ongoing account evaluations should provide accurate information on a payer's reimbursement behavior. This information is critical for supporting negotiations and evaluating the success of negotiation strategies. In payer negotiations, it is important to determine what can be negotiated and what is nonnegotiable.

For example, government-based payers usually do not negotiate with individual providers because payment policies are set through regulation. However, if a high percentage of bills are disputed, it may be important to determine the source of the problem. If, for example, the provider finds that there is a training problem with billing staff, the payer may be approached for training resources. Certainly the provider can appeal to the payer for assistance and resources to remedy an identified problem. In addition, revenue problems may be shared across a group of providers. Reimbursement policies for certain categories of procedures may need adjustment, and evidence from account evaluation can be extremely useful to support adjustment requests. In the case of government payers, such requests may enter the political arena, and state and federal elected officials may be requested to intervene. Professional associations such as the American Nurses Association, the Medical Group Management Association, and state-level professional organizations can become involved in reimbursement policy for providers. Special interest groups such as AARP can also be engaged in such discussions; it is often in the best interests of consumer groups to advocate for adequate provider reimbursement for necessary healthcare services. Consumer groups know that lack of adequate reimbursement for healthcare services results in shortages of service supply, and this is not in the best interests of either consumers or the providers who care for them. The importance of good evidence on the reimbursement of service providers cannot be overestimated in these situations. Therefore, reimbursement analysis and revenue evaluation are essential to support good healthcare reimbursement policy.

In the case of private payers, negotiation strategy must still involve the best possible evidence to show the cost basis for the level of quality care expected by healthcare consumers. A clear analysis of costs, reimbursement, and revenue form a solid basis for productive negotiation with a private payer. It is in the best interests of both providers and consumers to guarantee adequate reimbursement for healthcare services. It is also important for the provider to demonstrate control of overhead costs and careful management of the direct costs necessary to provide quality care. These subjects will be addressed in the following chapters.

## 7.6.  Concept Checkout

Be sure you understand these concepts before you begin the discussion questions:

- Reimbursement plan
- Operational revenue management
- Revenue cycle
- Revenue matching
- Balance billing
- Account management
- Revenue management cycle
- Revenue optimization
- Payer negotiation strategies

## 7.7.  Discussion Questions

1. Explain the relationship between the reimbursement plan and operational revenue management.
2. Outline the main strategies that might be used to match the receivables cycle with the payables cycle.
3. Research the balance billing regulations for one major payer. Include regulatory requirements, the penalties if regulations are not followed, and the revenue implications for the practice.
4. Research the strategies used by practice managers to optimize revenue management. You may want to interview a local practice manager to understand the practical implications of optimal revenue management.
5. List three main payer negotiation strategies and the evidence that you would use to support negotiations.

## 7.8.  References

Centers for Medicare and Medicaid Services. 2012. Medicare Secondary Payer for Provider, Physician, and Other Supplier Billing Staff. www.cms.gov/Outreach-and-

Education/Medicare-Learning-Network-MLN/MLNProducts/downloads/MSP_Fact_Sheet.pdf.

Mather, S. and K. Lorusso. 2012. "RCM, A Critical Component of Accountability Models: Revenue Cycle Management Holds the Key to Successful Financial Contracting in the World of Accountability Reform." *Health Management Technology* 33 (2): 26–27.

Nelson, B. 1994. "Improving Cash-Flow Through Benchmarking." *Healthcare Financial Management* 48:9: 74–78.

TripleTree. 2006. Healthcare Revenue Cycle Management: A TripleTree Industry Analysis. www.medicalmime.net/wp-content/uploads/2013/01/TripleTreeRevenueCycle-WhitePaper.pdf.

# CHAPTER 8

# Budgeting for Ambulatory Care Practices

## 8.1. Chapter Objectives

After completing the chapter you should be able to:

1. Define the relationship between strategic planning and budgeting.
2. List the main types of budgets and the steps for constructing them.
3. Analyze an existing expense budget and identify potential budget categories.
4. Explain the use of budget categories in constructing the chart of accounts.
5. Discuss the analysis of budget performance in the context of the goals of the firm.

## 8.2. Strategic Planning, Budgeting, and Budget Evaluation

The received wisdom that a budget is a strategic plan with a price tag provides a simple way of viewing the relationship between plans and budgets. At the start of any enterprise, the simple application of financial resources to the strategic vision might represent an organizational starting point. However, in most cases the relationship between plans and budgets in healthcare organizations is more subtle and complex. We have seen that in ambulatory care the relationship between strategic plan and budget is moderated by both external and internal influences. This section presents a brief discussion of some of the main factors on the ambulatory care planning and budgeting process.

*The business strategy of the practice in a given health environment is a major budgetary influence.* Business strategy is affected by the skills and abilities of the principals in the practice, their values and beliefs about healthcare, and the environment surrounding the enterprise. One of the most important features of the practice environment is the health status of the population in the area the practice serves and the provider's beliefs about the relationship between healthcare and health. Historically the delivery of ambulatory care was seen as a response to illness. The promotion of wellness, while supported theoretically, was not emphasized in practice nor expected by the consumer. Research supports this point. For example, a study of the treatment of smoking during ambulatory visits from 1994 to 2003 (Thorndike, Regan, and Rigotti, 2006), showed that counseling against smoking, a well-established health risk, occurred in only 20 percent of smokers' primary care visits in the years 2001–2003, and in 22 percent of smokers' visits in 1994–1996. While the reasons for this finding have not been definitively established, researchers postulate that it may be due to the lack of reimbursement for smoking-cessation counseling during the period studied. However, the variation in the provision of this service certainly reflects differing views of the need to use practice resources to support preventive care. For the 20 percent of the practices that did provide counseling, it might be assumed that the strategic use of resources was influenced by the practitioner's value for preventive care, as all practices faced a similar reimbursement environment.

*The reimbursement environment* in which a practice operates impacts on both strategic planning and budgetary allocations. As the above smoking research suggests, the fact that a preventive service is not paid for makes it highly unlikely that a practice will allocate resources for it. The reimbursement environment also influences the relative weight placed on various activities within the practice. Highly profitable services are likely to be prioritized in the practice's business strategy, while services that are costly to produce and less profitable to deliver are less emphasized.

Economists argue that markets express their preferences through pricing: providers are willing to prioritize relatively profitable services while individuals are willing to pay a higher price for services that they value more. We have seen that in healthcare market forces are quite distorted; an individual's demand in particular is distorted by lack of information about the comparative quality and health benefit of specific services, as well as by the presence of a third-party payer that takes the burden of direct payment off the patient's shoulders while steering patients toward or away from certain services. The inevitable conclusion is that strategic planning and budgeting does not wholly reflect the strategic vision or values of the practice owners or the response of the consumers to their own health needs. The strategy a practice defines and to which it allocates resources may reflect the reimbursement decisions of a third-party payer, whose decisions are made largely to manage the payer's risk.

*Consumer preference* may shape strategic planning and budgeting within the practice, but responding to these preferences is not direct. Consumers express their market preferences in ambulatory healthcare by selecting a provider. The influence of the third-party payer and the regulator is clearly seen in this area of the healthcare market. For example, providers need to be included in a payers' panel in order to be selected by the consumer. If they are not in the payers' panel, consumers may visit them, but they will pay more out of pocket to do so. This distorts the price-to-value equation for the consumer because a portion of what the consumer pays does not reflect absolute value for the service provided but rather a penalty. The consumer may be willing to pay this penalty for several reasons: (1) he or she distrusts the providers in the panel sufficiently to seek care outside or (2) he or she highly values the provider and willingly pays the penalty. In either case, the relationship between price and consumer value is distorted by the out-of-network penalty. A provider trying to strategically position a practice with consumers cannot simply focus on providing care that appeals most to patients. Providers must also consider the additional step of either joining a payer's panel, elevating their value with consumers to a level that considers the out-of-network penalty, or simply providing an alternative source of care to consumers who want to opt out of the panel. Providers seeking to influence consumer choice need to consider costs beyond the price-value equation for services.

As the above discussion illustrates, a practice's strategic planning and budget decisions are not a mirror reflection of its business preferences and values. These decisions are also shaped by reimbursement practices and consumer preferences, which are prone to distortions due to incomplete information and third-party roles.

## 8.3. Constructing Budgets: A Focus on Revenue and Expense

Unless the practice is new, budgets are typically constructed based on past budgets. As the previous discussion has shown, the practice would be well advised to review not only its own strategic vision but also the reimbursement environment and consumer preferences in its service area before following exactly the budgets of the previous period.

There are two operational budgetary documents: the revenue budget and the expense budget. The *revenue budget* is based on the revenue planning tools we have previously discussed: the reimbursement analysis, which focuses on the payer environment, and the revenue analysis, which focuses on reimbursement sources within the practice. These two analytical tools provide the practice with the information required to compile the annual revenue budget and to forecast revenues for a longer-term revenue budget. While some lenders or other regulators may require a 10- or 15-year revenue budget projection, most experienced healthcare financial planners will say that a five-year horizon is the most that can be considered realistic or reliable in the current heathcare climate. The changing technology, labor force, and reimbursement strategies in healthcare create a lack of stability that makes long-term planning unreliable.

Construction of the revenue budget is a straightforward process of listing all expected sources of revenue, the number of service units expected to be delivered, and the revenue expected from each service unit. Some financial-management sources suggest that the volume estimates be prepared as a separate document called a volume budget that defines the level of utilization by reimbursement category. This is useful when almost all revenue is earned on a fee-for-service basis. Practices that receive some capitated payments may find the volume budget useful to calculate expense, but is not helpful to understand revenue that is based on the negotiated payment for the group. The format of the revenue budget is shown in Figure 8.1. This budget reflects a practice that receives some fee-for-service revenue and some capitated payments. Performance analysis of the revenue budget defined in this way has to consider volume variances to understand month-to-month revenue variances for the Blue Cross payer but not as much for the capitated payer because intrayear enrollment is mostly steady. This will be discussed in more detail in the section on budget analysis.

Revenue Budget for Period ____1/1____ to ____1/31____

| Payer | Projected Volume | Revenue/unit | Total Revenue |
|---|---|---|---|
| Blue Cross | 100 < =15-minute visits | $ 60.00/visit | $6,000 |
| Blue Cross | 100 < =30-minute visits | $ 80.00/visit | $8,000 |
| Blue Cross | 100 < =45-minute visits | $100.00/visit | $10,000 |
| Capitation | 100 members | $ 100 pmpm | $16,000 |

*FIGURE 8.1. Revenue budget format.*

*Expense budgets* are usually constructed using historical data corrected for inflation and changes in practice labor, supplies, technology, and physical plant. As with revenue budgets, the projection of expenses out farther than five years in expense budgets is difficult and largely unreliable. To be accurate, expense budgets should always consider variations in volume and input prices. Variances from the budgeted level of expense may be driven by an unexpected change in the volume of services delivered, an increase in the prices paid for labor, material, or technology, or a provider shift toward more resource-intensive methods. Accurate understanding of the variance drivers is important if expenses are to be managed appropriately. This is particularly relevant when practices are paid on a capitated basis and the revenue received for services is a flat monthly rate. If the expense of providing care exceeds revenue, the practice must accurately pinpoint the reason if it is to remain in business. The nature of the expenses is also important to consider. Chapter 6 provides an in-depth discussion of costs and cost behavior that is important to understand before an expense budget is created.

## 8.4.  Expense Budgets and Categories

A new practice faces a difficult challenge when creating its first expense budget. In this case it is important to review the costing information presented in Chapter 6 and conduct a careful cost analysis that provides the basis for the first expense budget. The main cost drivers in a primary care practice are labor, supplies, and equipment. It is also important to understand the costs of acquiring and maintaining the facility in which the practice is located. A practice usually negotiates a rental package that includes basic facility and grounds maintenance, security, and janitorial services. Extra costs can include specialized maintenance of plumbing and other utilities required by the practice technology, disposal of hazardous waste to comply with regulations, and the specialized cleaning required in a medical facility. A careful analysis of these additional maintenance costs is important to create an accurate budget and avoid unexpected costs. Changes in the regulations that pertain to medical practices should also be carefully monitored to ensure compliance for a business license. Expenses related to the license renewal need to be considered also.

A participatory approach to creating and reviewing the expense budget categories is important because the expectations of the partners and staff need to be understood. For example, professionals employed by the practice may expect the practice to assist them with professional licensure or membership fees, conference travel, professional journal subscriptions or publication fees. The practice may wish to accommodate these requests, but it must consider carefully the expense level that can be included in the budget. A strategic discussion with the practice professionals prior to the new budget year prevents later budgetary pressures that might not be easily accommodated. This is particularly true for large professional expenses such as personal malpractice coverage, specialty licensure, or license renewal. The development of expense policies in a participatory manner prevents later disputes and dissatisfaction. Participation of staff in expense-budget planning helps them understand efficient office management. Frequently staff is unaware of the cost of expendable supplies or variable labor. Increasing the staff's understanding of the relationship between controlling expenses, on the one hand, and bonuses paid out of net revenue, on the other, generally results in more attention to efficiency and control of costs.

In general, the definition of budget categories in a new practice depends on the cost analysis together with participatory discussions with the practice staff. For established practices, examination of the historical expense record and discussion with practice staff is the best way to arrive at expense categories for the new budget.

## 8.5.  Building a Chart of Accounts

A new practice needs to build a chart of accounts that organizes its assets, liabilities, expenses, and revenues. A chart of accounts is simply a numbered list of the categories of financial transactions the practice is likely to use. The chart includes real accounts that are cumulative records of financial transactions in respective categories since the inception of the business, and nominal accounts that are closed at the end of every fiscal year. Nominal accounts typically include revenues and expenses while real accounts include assets, liabilities, and owners' equity. At the end of the fiscal year, the revenue and expense accounts are finalized, expenses are subtracted from revenue, and the net operating margin is moved to the owner's or partners' equity account. The nominal accounts are closed and a new accounting period begins.

The practice principals and their financial manager should review the list of nominal accounts at the end of each fiscal year to determine the adequacy of the accounts for the next period. At this point they may wish to add, remove, regroup, or redefine revenue or expense accounts that no longer reflect the anticipated cash flow in the business. This review of nominal accounts ensures that the chart reflects current business practice in both revenue and expenses. The chart organizes the way that revenue and expenses are reported so that data is placed in a context that allows precise practice management through evaluation of financial performance.

## 8.6.  Evaluating Budget Performance: Goal Achievement

The annual financial performance goals of a practice depend on following the budget targets defined at the start of the fiscal year. Budget performance is examined through variance analysis, which compares the budget target to the actual financial performance and calculates the difference. Ambulatory care organizations should always define revenue and expense targets using a flexible budget approach for fee-for-service payers. Because the majority of ambulatory services delivered in the United States are reimbursed at fee-for-service rates, most practices should gather cost and revenue data by unit of care delivered and create a relative value scale (RVU) for use in budgeting. The steps for creating this scale depend on a definition of the basic service unit for the practice. Here are the steps to creating the RVU: (1) Define the basic unit of service, which is the smallest unit of service that can be on a bill. For example, a brief office visit, lasting about 15 minutes, might be the basic service unit in a primary care practice. (2) Allocate costs to this basic unit in the major categories of labor, supplies, technology, and allocated indirect costs. (3) Project how many basic units will be delivered in the next budget period. (4) Determine the budget for the period by multiplying the cost of the basic units by the projected number.

Once it defines the cost of an RVU (Example 8.1), the practice

---

### Example 8.1—RVU Development

The basic unit of service is a 15-minute office visit. The cost of this visit includes as follows:

a. Provider's time
b. Supplies such as sterile and non-sterile material and drugs.
c. Technology use, such as diagnostic laboratory and the visit's share of depreciated capital cost of equipment, repair, and mainenance.
d. Allocated indirect costs that include standard overhead items.

| | |
|---|---|
| Provider's Time | $ 30.00 |
| Supplies | $  7.00 |
| Technology | $ 10.00 |
| Indirect Costs | $  6.00 |
| **Total Cost/RVU** | **$ 53.00** |

| Example 8.2—RVUs Delivered in 1 Month | | |
|---|---|---|
| | | #RVUs |
| 1400 brief visits | ≤ 15 min | 1400 |
| 800 intermediate | ≤ 30 min | 1600 |
| 550 complex | ≤ 45 min | 1650 |
| **Total RVUs delivered** | | **4650** |

should examine historical data and current contracts to estimate the number of RVUs to be delivered. Additionally, the practice should project the allowed charge per RVU to assess revenue from the fee-for-service payer. For capitated payers, estimate expenses for RVUs, but revenue will depend on the negotiated flat payment per enrolled patient. A simple multiplication of the number of projected RVUs by the cost or revenue per RVU gives the expense and revenue target figures. Note that the RVU expense can be disaggregated into its components for management purposes. The expense budget can then be examined in four areas: direct labor, supplies, technology, and allocated indirect costs. This disaggregation provides useful information for direct management of budgets. In Example 8.2, a practice has categorized clinic visits using a 15-minute visit as the basic RVU. Intermediate visits lasting between 16 and 30 minutes are allocated 2 RVUs, and complex visits are 3 RVUs. Patient encounter data from electronic medical records systems shows that 4650 RVUs were delivered in one month.

Once you know the total RVUs delivered for the month, a simple calculation determines the budget variance: subtract the amount budgeted from the amount spent.

Table 8.1 illustrates the advantage of disaggregating the total costs into cost categories. Suggested areas for management to investigate include the use of provider's time and the technology cost. The overrun in indirect costs does not require intense management attention,

TABLE 8.1. One-Month Budget for Ambulatory Care Practice.

| Cost Category | RVU | Actual | Budget | Variance |
|---|---|---|---|---|
| Provider's Time | $ 30.00 | $ 170,000 | $ 139,500 | ($30,500) |
| Technology Cost | $ 10.00 | $  50,000 | $  46,500 | ($3,500) |
| Supply Cost | $  7.00 | $  25,000 | $  32,550 | $7,550 |
| Indirects | $  6.00 | $  28,000 | $  27,900 | ($100) |
| Total | $ 53.00 | $ 273,000 | $  46,450 | ($26,550) |

although an analysis of the origin of the negative variance would be beneficial. Priority attention needs to be directed to the use of provider time if the practice is to remain solvent.

Strategic variance analysis may also be an important area for management attention. For example, if the practice has defined increased use of registered nurses for patient education about medication management, determine if the variance in the cost of provider's time is due to more RN time or more MD time. If the variance is due to the increase in RN time, it may be important to address how education is being conducted rather than simply mandating less of it. If the increase is in MD time, then it might be useful to understand if RNs are involved in the patient visit at all and if the strategic objective is being achieved. While drilling down in the area of the largest observed variance the manager needs to consider not only the fact that the budget was overspent but also the strategic mandates and whether they were achieved.

## 8.7.  Concept Checkout

Be sure you understand these concepts before you begin the discussion questions:

- The relationship between strategic planning and budgeting
- Influences on the planning and budgeting processes
- Revenue budget
- Expense budget
- Chart of accounts
- Real accounts
- Nominal accounts
- Relative value units
- Variance analysis
- Strategic variance analysis

## 8.8.  Discussion Questions

1. As a new practice administrator in an existing practice, describe the steps you will take to become familiar with the budgeting process.
2. You discover that the practice does not use RVUs because 60 percent of its revenue is capitated. Design a brief staff in-service to explain the reasons that RVUs are important despite the flat reimbursements.
3. You are one month away from the end of the fiscal year and are

discussing the annual budget cycle with your accounting firm. You have noticed that some of the accounts listed in the chart of accounts are never used. What questions do you need to ask about these accounts, and what steps would you recommend to the accountant?

4. In reviewing the latest variance report you noticed a large negative variance in technology costs that is completely offset by a large positive variance in labor costs. What steps would you recommend to the practice manager?

5. You are working in a practice that is 100 percent owned by a capitated payer, and you receive a flat monthly payment to take care of the 50,000 patients registered to your practice. You have only a small staff. Would you recommend establishing an RVU system? Why or why not?

## 8.9. Reference

Thorndike, Anne N., Susan Regan, and Nancy A. Rigotti. 2007. "The Treatment of Smoking by US Physicians during Ambulatory Visits: 1994–2003." *American Journal of Public Health* 97 (10): 1878–83.

# New Day Health and Associates

*You should not attempt this case, which requires significant market research, until you have completed Chapters 1–8 in your textbook.*

You are an experienced family nurse practitioner, and you have decided to join with three colleagues to open a primary-care practice called New Day Health and Associates. The practice will focus on health rather than acute care. You and your colleagues strongly believe that patient teaching, health promotion, and careful attention to families and individuals with chronic health problems can decrease the cost of care and increase quality of life for your clients. You have incorporated your practice as a 501(c)(3) organization so that you could invest your net revenue in a public health cause, for example to support the Healthy People 2020 activities in your state. This implies that you must be particularly budget-conscious because you will not carry over funds to cushion your practice in difficult times.

When selecting a location for the practice, be sure to review demographic data, and do not select a location for which there is none available. The more demographic and provider data you have, the easier it will be to do a good case analysis.

Answer the following questions. You will need to do some research and reading to answer them adequately.

1. How will you determine the market area that you are going to serve? List at least three strategic considerations in picking a location.
2. Describe at least two major payers in your market. They can be

public or private payers. Provide information on how they pay for care (fee for service, discounted fee for service, capitation, or partial capitation).

3. Discuss the linkage between strategic planning and budgeting for your first year of practice. Provide at least two examples with details on how you will link your budget to your care-delivery strategy.

4. Provide a detailed outline of the revenue analysis of the two payers you identified in question 2. Highlight the impact of your business strategy on the type of revenue analysis you do for each payer.

5. Present a sample revenue budget for one health education service based on the two payers you have identified. Your budget should be quantified using RVUs.

6. Present a sample expense budget for the health education service identified in question 5. Remember to include expenses consistent with your strategic plan for patient care.

7. Present an initial proposal for nominal accounts to be used in your chart of accounts for the health education services you intend to provide. Your nominal accounts will be revenue and expense accounts. Provide a proposal for the accounts you will need in both of these areas.

8. Outline the monthly variance report you will request from your accounting firm for the health education services you have analyzed in the previous questions. Provide a discussion of what you will do with the variance report after you receive it.

# Section 5

# CHAPTER 9

# Capitalization Structure and Investment Planning

## 9.1. Chapter Objectives

After completing the chapter you should be able to:

1. Define the term capital structure.
2. Discuss the implications of capital structure for the patient care practice.
3. Analyze the effect of taxes on capital structure.
4. Define the effect of risk on capital structure.
5. Discuss capital structure planning in the context of a patient care practice.

## 9.2. Capitalization Structure Planning

Capital structure is the mix of debt and equity financing a business needs to accomplish its strategic mission. In a healthcare practice, capital structure planning starts with its strategic plan, the owner's roadmap of services that the practice will offer, the payers it expects to work with, and the amount of third-party insurance payment involved. An evidence-based, feasible practice strategy is essential for sound capital-structure planning. Once the practice has defined its strategy it can assess the costs associated with start-up and the first-year financial requirements. Start-up costs include acquiring fixed assets such as medical equipment, office property, office furniture, and systems for billing, medical records, practice management, accounting, and communications. Start-up analysis also must consider staffing levels and the amount of wages that will need to be paid before any revenue is received. Additional costs associated with the start-up period include those for establishing business ownership and governance structure, start-up accounting, business licenses and permits, affiliation and hospital credentialing, and malpractice coverage, which may include coverage for providers joining from other practices that did not provide "tail-claim" coverage. Many practices hire consultants to assist them in managing these start-up complexities. Consultants can also assist with strategic planning, or they may only focus on the mechanics of establishing a practice that has already defined a strategy. In either case, funds for consultant fees should be included as an expense when planning capital structure.

The sources of funds define the initial capital structure of the practice. If a practice decides to borrow to cover start-up costs, it is important to identify investors of equity capital because lenders usually do not consider a start-up proposal without capital from investors. The conditions under which the investor provides capital will concern any lender because the investor's expectations and rights impact the practice in many ways. For example, if an investor expects some voice in governance or a limit to the amount of debt, these expectations should be agreed to before the investor's funds are accepted. If the practice owners are the primary investors, careful discussion should still occur so that all owner-investors are satisfied with the management strategy and agreements. Practice ownership, governance, compensation, and profit-sharing arrangements all need to be defined carefully. Failure to do so can lead to serious situations later, particularly if the practice's finances present challenges for the partners to resolve.

## 9.3.  The Effect of Capitalization Structure on Performance

The total financial requirements to start a practice are met with investment funds and some borrowed funds. The ratio of borrowed to investment funds defines the practice's capital structure. Once the level of debt is established, a source of borrowed funds must be identified. In order to qualify for a business loan, a practice must meet the prospective lenders' requirement of a clear strategic plan, a set of pro-forma financial statements, a one-year budget, and a business plan. Lenders also look favorably on financial investment by the practice owners because it signals seriousness of purpose and responsibility for the outcome. If personal funds are not available, outside investors may sometimes be attracted by consulting sources of venture capital or government subsidies for practitioners willing to locate in underserved areas. A personal loan to the practice owners rather than to the business entity is another possible source of investment capital. This option generally requires personal collateral, such as equity in a home or other property or value. If no collateral is available a personal loan may still be possible, but the interest rate will likely be high and the term of the loan short. If owners take this route for initial investment capital, it increases income requirements because the owners must include loan payments as a personal expense. This increases the start-up finance requirements of the practice as a business entity.

The ratio of borrowed to invested funds that defines the capital structure is called the debt/equity (or debt-to-equity) ratio. A debt/equity ratio of 1 indicates that for every dollar invested, the practice has borrowed one dollar. Lenders analyze industry standards and current economic conditions to decide the debt-to-equity ratio they will accept in a loan application. In periods of economic recession, lenders prefer lower ratios than in the time of economic growth, when higher debt-to-equity ratios are acceptable.

In general, the assumption of debt increases the practice's production efficiency requirement. This is sometimes called the discipline of debt. Because an external lender places repayment requirements on the practice, the practice must earn sufficient income to repay the lender and also cover practice expenses. The discipline of debt increases the practice's attention to effective and efficient management so it meets repayment requirements. The risks of debt are also obvious; in seeking to maximize the volume of billable services, the practice may compromise the quality of care.

At the start of any practice, careful consideration needs to be given to the debt capacity the practice believes it has in relation to the strategy it has defined. Exceeding this debt capacity creates a significant risk of poor practice performance financially and in the quality of care for its patients.

This discussion highlights the necessity to locate not only willing lenders but also investors willing to provide funds to capitalize the practice. The least preferred option is investment capital obtained through personal debt of the practice owners. Every effort should be made to avoid this scenario by identifying external sources of investment capital.

## 9.4.  The World of Taxation and Its Effects on Capital

The capital structure decision must also consider the impact of tax deductibility on the use of debt or equity. All else equal, there is a tax advantage to the use of debt in the capital structure of a business because interest payments on business debt are tax deductible as long as they are treated as business expenses. This provides a tax advantage to practices that include debt in their capital structure. However, as previous discussion has shown, there are other considerations in this decision. For example, equity holders generally expect a return on their investment, and the practice needs to ensure that it can service debt and still provide some return on invested capital. That is why the decision between using debt and equity must consider return on investment planning as well as the favorable tax treatment of debt. Equity holders generally have many choices when considering investments. They expect to earn a return at least equal to other options they could have chosen. A practice that provides no return to equity partners may face withdrawal of capital by investors. Replacing investors' capital may force the practice partners to incur unplanned debt, which is usually more expensive and harder to obtain than planned debt. Careful planning of capital structure leads to a balanced capitalization that both supports equity holders and allows for timely interest payments to debt holders. Planning should also consider the tax implications of using debt in the capital structure as well as the equity holders' expectations of return on investment.

There are other taxation considerations to address in capital structure planning, particularly for providers who enter the practice with significant student loan debt. Since the interest on student loan debt is not tax deductible, the practice needs to consider the income expectations of the indebted healthcare professional as well as options to reduce or eliminate student loan debt. For example, there may be state or federal student loan forgiveness in places lacking healthcare services, and practices may be able to assist potential providers to obtain this subsidy. This has clear advantages for the practice because income expectations may be lowered if a potential employee's student loan debt can be eliminated. Recent research shows that the average debt of U.S. medical-school graduates is more than $170,000 (American Association of Medical Colleges, 2013). Repayment scenarios for physicians vary depending on their time in residency programs and their employment choices after training is completed. But under any scenario, repayment takes at least ten years at varying proportions of after-tax income (American Association of Medical Colleges, 2013). A similar situation also pertains to nurse practitioners, who generally enter graduate school at mid-career and incur a higher opportunity cost of their education (earnings foregone during the years of graduate education). These graduates expect sufficient income to repay student loan debt and the opportunity cost of their education. Enabling forgiveness of non-tax-deductible student loan debt significantly impacts income expectations of both nurse practitioners and physicians.

Part of the capital structure planning for the practice might also be use of some tax-deductible business debt to help practice partners pay interest on their student loan debt. Interest payments are a deductible business expense for the practice, but not for the individual practitioners. So there may be financial advantage to subsidizing student loan repayment if loan forgiveness cannot be obtained. Analysis of the tax and business expense implications of these options is important given the current tax advantages for corporate debt and the high personal indebtedness of the practice partners.

## 9.5.  Risk and Capitalization

There are two categories of risk to consider when planning capital structure: business risk and financial risk. Uncertainty results in external and internal business risk. Payment reforms, government regulations, and changes in disease trends stipulate external business risk. Uncertainty created by new technology like electronic medical records or diagnostic tools can lead to internal business risk. Financial risk often ensues from capital structure decisions such as the level of debt, the expectations of equity partners, and changes in taxation policy. Financial risk also results from changes in financial policies of insurers and suppliers, and from stress on employees about changing financial conditions within the practice.

In general, financial uncertainty increases financial risk. The higher the levels of debt in the capital structure the greater the uncertainty of repayment capacity. This is why highly leveraged practices (those operating at a high debt-to-equity ratio) must pay higher interest rates when they take on more debt financing. Every unit increase in debt raises the uncertainty as to whether the practice can meet its repayment responsibilities; this uncertainty is translated into a risk-premium levied by lenders when additional debt is requested. Equity holders make a risk calculation about a practice, just as they do about a return on investment. If an equity holder (external to practice partners) deems a practice a poor long-term investment, the holder requires a higher short-term return. If it does not receive that return, it withdraws the investment capital, which increases the risk profile for the remaining investors and results in higher interest rates. It is easy to see that managing both financial and business risk lowers practice financial costs (costs to access capital).

Information is a key component of financial- and business-risk management (Paterson and Wendel, 1996). Careful use of business intelligence coupled with good use of financial data to shape capital structure decisions lowers risk profile and costs. Practices that invest in pertinent data and use it wisely increase efficiency and lower financial and business risk.

## 9.6.  Capital Structure Planning for the Primary Care Provider

Primary healthcare is delivered in an organizational framework in which providers are given access to the technology, staff, and supplies. This organizational structure requires financial capital to support its establishment and sustained operation. Planning the capital structure for primary care requires a feasible organizational strategy, understanding of the external environment, and information to assess the business and financial risks facing the practice. The assessment of internal organizational strengths, weaknesses, opportunities, and threats (SWOT) is a widely used planning framework to support capital structure planning.

Internal organizational strengths and weaknesses should include both business and financial risk assessment. The practice's management experience and expertise, healthcare technology, and provider availability and experience need to be assessed before making capital structure decisions. For example, a practice in a highly competitive labor market may have personnel who need access to labor-substituting technology because labor is both scarce and expensive. Conversely, in less competitive labor markets, the practice has more staff and needs less costly technology because labor is available at a more affordable cost. The internal organization of these practices suggests different capital requirements and allocations; one may face larger fixed costs for expensive labor and technology while the other may be able to manage with more variable labor costs and less technology. To allocate capital wisely, a practice should conduct an evidence-based evaluation of its preferred mix of labor and technology.

The external environment has a major influence on capital structure planning. The current emphasis on electronic medical records by public and private payers is an excellent example of this. By 2015, Medicare will require the meaningful use of certified electronic medical record systems by all providers who submit bills. Providers unable to meet this deadline will pay increasing penalties for noncompliance (http://www.medicalrecords.com/physicians/electronic-medical-records-deadline). The cost of acquiring such a system ranges from $10,000 to $32,600, according to a recent cost-benefit study (Wang *et al.*, 2012). Medicare's regulatory decisions confer capital costs on primary care practices. Providers who do not gather environmental information before finalizing the capital structure plan may face larger unplanned costs and increased financial risks during their start-up phase. As we have seen, increased financial risk results in higher borrowing and equity costs that impact efficiency and quality. The use of information to assess internal and external conditions is vital for optimal capital structure planning.

While many providers rely on financial consultants to conduct a SWOT analysis and recommend the capitalization structure, there is no substitute for involvement by the practice principals in this planning process. We have seen that a high level of technical understanding is required to assess the practice's operational strengths and challenges. Most financial consultants rely on the practice owners to provide this information and assess the impact of internal capacity on the capital structure decisions. Consultants can reasonably be expected to supply an analysis of the taxation environment, the general practices of lenders, the expectations of investors, and the financial regulatory situation. However, this knowledge is not complete until it is added to a clear and realistic appraisal of the practice capacities, labor, and technology needs. External consultants should never make the final capital structure decision alone, and it is seldom wise to make this critical decision without some consideration of expert opinion external to the practice. As in many financial planning situations, optimal evidence-based decisions are made after analysis and consultation with appropriate experts, on the one hand, and realistic internal assessments of practice capability, on the other.

## 9.7. Concept Checkout

Be sure you understand these concepts before you begin the discussion questions:

- Capital structure
- Total financial requirements
- Start-up costs
- Equity
- Debt
- Debt-to-equity ratio
- Discipline of debt
- Business risk
- Financial risk
- Risk premium
- SWOT analysis

## 9.8. Discussion Questions

1. You have decided to open a primary care practice in New York City focused on serving the Medicaid population. List three initial questions you need to consider to plan your capital structure.
2. You decide that you will accept a high level of debt to open your

practice. List at least two potential risks the practice will face due to this capitalization decision.

3. Three of the four partners in this incorporated practice have more than $150,000 in student loan debt. Discuss at least two implications the practice faces from this level of personal indebtedness.

4. One of the partners was employed by another primary care practice in the city for the last five years. Discuss one major start-up financial consideration for this partner joining the practice.

5. At your first start-up partners' meeting, one of the nurse practitioners said he did not want to be involved in making a capital structure recommendation. He wanted to leave it to the financial professionals at your bank to recommend the level of debt and investment required. Formulate a reaction to this statement and provide a rationale for your own recommendation in response to this partner.

## 9.9. References

American Association of Medical Colleges. 2013. "Physician Education Debt and the Cost to Attend Medical School: 2012 Update." www.aamc.org/download/328322/data/statedebtreport.pdf.

Paterson, M. and J. Wendel. 1996. "Managing Risk in a Changing Health Care System." *Journal of Health Care Finance* 22: 15–22.

Wang, S. J., B. Middleton, L. A. Prosser, C. G. Bardon, C. D. Spurr, P. J. Carchidi, A. F. Kittler, R. C. Goldszer, D. G. Fairchild, A. J. Sussman, G. J. Kuperman, D. W. Bates. 2003. "A cost-benefit analysis of electronic medical records in primary care." *American Journal of Medicine.* 114(5): 396–403.

# CHAPTER 10

# Basic Financial Statements

## 10.1. Chapter Objectives

After completing the chapter you should be able to:

1. State the purpose of each of the four basic financial statements.
2. Explain how the balance sheet is related to the income and expense statement.
3. Define the elements of the cash flow statement and identify its relationship to the balance sheet.
4. Explain the relationship of financial statements to financial ratios.

## 10.2. The Four Basic Financial Reports

Financial performance is represented in standardized reports that provide information to internal managers and to external stakeholders. In healthcare, external stakeholders include lenders, investors, and regulators, all of whom require knowledge of the financial state and prospects of a healthcare practice. Lenders are primarily interested in the capacity of a practice to repay debt; investors want to assess the prospects of a fair return on their invested capital; and regulators act to represent the public's interests in the practice's capacity for quality care at an affordable price in compliance with the tax, licensing, and quality requirements of the government. Each of these stakeholders requires diverse information that is usually provided in four basic financial reports. These reports are commonly prepared by accounting professionals who can certify that the documents comply with generally accepted accounting principles that have been codified by the Financial Accounting Standards Board (FASB)—most recently in 2008. Currently the FASB is working with the International Accounting Standards Board toward a set of converged principles that apply to both U.S. and international businesses. The purpose of standardization of accounting practices is to communicate clearly to a range of financial and non-financial managers, investors, and regulators about the status of a business. Standardization also allows comparisons regarding the relative position of a business among its competitors and assessing average financial performance across similar firms.

There are three standardized reports that represent aspects of the business and one report that shows changes in investor's interests in the business over a period of time. The three basic financial reports about the business include (1) a report of business assets and how they are financed at a given point in time (the balance sheet); (2) a report on how much money the business earned and spent over a defined time period (the income and expense statement); and (3) an accounting of how money flowed between the business and the external environment (the cash flow statement). Practice owners and managers need to understand the purpose, organization, and sources of required data for each report. The fourth report, which documents changes in shareholders' (i.e., investors') equity, is important because, as we have seen, investment capital is essential to a practice, particularly during the start-up phase. Table 10.1 summarizes the four reports.

## 10.3. Putting the Financial Picture Together: The Interaction of the Income and Expense Statement and the Balance Sheet

To understand the interaction of these financial reports, we will discuss the preparation of the annual income and expense report (otherwise named profit and loss (P&L) report or statement) and the balance sheet. The practice owners look first at the "bottom line" of the income and expense statement, which is the net revenue earned after all the expenses and taxes have been paid over a specified period of time. Net revenue is the last line of the income and expense report, as shown in Figure 10.1.

You can see from the organization of this report that it must cover a specific period of time, for example one year. Most practice managers and owners review profit and loss statements regularly to be sure that there are no serious revenue or expense problems developing in the practice. Notice that the profit and loss statement does not report accounts receivable as a separate category.

The notes accompanying the profit and loss statement would doc-

TABLE 10.1. *Summary of Financial Reports.*

| Report | Purpose | Basic Formula | Data Sources |
|---|---|---|---|
| Income and expense report, also called profit and loss (P&L) report. | Shows how much revenue the business earned and the resources it required over a defined time period. | Revenues − expenses = net income (profit) for the defined period. | General ledger: All revenue and expense accounts, including tax accounts. |
| Balance sheet, or statement of financial position. | A snapshot of the business's financial condition at a particular point in time. | Assets = liabilities + equity at a point in time. | General ledger: All asset, liability, and equity accounts. |
| Cash flow (or funds flow) statement. | Explains how a company raised and spent money over a defined period of time. | Net change in cash for a defined period = [net income + increases in liability − increases in assets] for the defined period. | Indirect method adjusts the net income from the profit and loss statement by deducting increases in general ledger asset accounts from net income and adding increases in general ledger liability accounts to net income for the reported period. |
| Statement of shareholders' or owners' equity. In publicly traded companies it is always called statement of shareholders' equity. | Explains the gains and losses in owners' or shareholders' equity over a defined period of time. | Change in owners' equity = change in invested capital (reported by class of stock in publicly traded companies) + change in retained earnings. | General ledger equity accounts for each class of stock, including capital stock owned by the business, general ledger account for retained earnings, and any other general ledger equity accounts. |

125

| Category | Amount in dollars |
|---|---|
| **Operating Revenue** | |
| Direct Patient Services | 700,000 |
| Health Promotion Counseling and Classes | 200,000 |
| Prisoners Health Contract | 100,000 |
| **Total Operating Revenue** | 1,000,000 |
| **Operating Expenses** | **1,000,000** |
| **Direct costs** | |
| Salaries | 300,000 |
| Contract labor | 100,000 |
| Supplies including stock pharmaceuticals | 75,000 |
| *Sub-total—direct costs* | *475,000* |
| **Indirect costs** | |
| Mortgage Payment | 80,000 |
| Insurance | 50,000 |
| Utilities | 30,000 |
| *Sub-total—indirect costs* | *160,000* |
| **Total Costs (direct + indirect costs)** | **635,000** |
| **NET REVENUE FROM OPERATIONS** | **365,000** |
| (Total Operating Revenue minus Total Costs) | |
| **Other Income (Expenses)** | |
| Loan Interest paid | (80,000) |
| Earnings Before Taxes | 285,000 |
| Income Taxes | (42,750) |
| Business Taxes | (12,000) |
| **NET REVENUE** | **230,250** |

**FIGURE 10.1.**   *The Income and Expense Report for General Practice Affiliates for Year XXXX.*

ument the accounting basis for the reports. If the firm reports on an accrual basis, revenue is considered received when it is billed, not when it is paid. Expenses are recognized when they are incurred, not when they are paid. If the firm keeps its accounts on a cash basis, then expenses and revenues are recognized when they are paid rather than billed. Healthcare practices vary in their selection of accounting basis, but you can understand the importance of knowing which basis is being used in order to appreciate the context of the profit and loss statement. In a firm that operates on an accrual basis, managers use the profit and loss statement together with the cash flow statement and balance sheet to understand the accounts receivable situation. For healthcare practices a clear picture of accounts receivable is very important. So if the practice accounting is on an accrual basis, regular review of balance sheets and cash flow analyses are also a critical part of the financial management system. If the firm is on a cash basis, there are problems matching revenues to the time period in which they are earned and in tracking billed services. In healthcare the accrual system is preferred because few services are paid for at the time they are delivered. Tracking accounts receivable is a major part of a healthcare financial manager's portfolio. Our discussion will focus on financial reports based on an accrual method because it provides essential information to the practice owners and managers.

The balance sheet presents a snapshot of a business's financial condition at a specified point in time. As Figure 10.2 shows, it can be generated at the start of a firm's fiscal year.

The balance sheet is organized according to the basic accounting equation:

$$assets = liabilities + equity$$

In the example, you can see that the practice had \$464,700 in assets. These assets were equal to \$53,400 in current liabilities plus \$20,000

| Assets | | Liabilities and Owners' Equity | |
|---|---|---|---|
| **Current Assets** | | **Current Liabilities** | |
| Cash | 2,100 | Accounts Payable | 35,900 |
| Petty Cash | 100 | Interest on Debt | 2,900 |
| Certificate of Deposit | 10,000 | Wages Payable | 8,500 |
| Accounts Receivable | 40,500 | Taxes Payable | 6,100 |
| Inventory | 31,000 | | |
| **Long-term Assets** | | **Long-term Liabilities and Equity** | |
| Property | 180,000 | Mortgage | 20,000 |
| Equipment | 201,000 | Owner's Equity | 161,050 |
| | | Retained Earnings | 230,250 |
| **TOTAL ASSETS** | **464,700** | **TOTAL LIABILITIES + EQUITY** | **464,700** |

**FIGURE 10.2.** *General Practice Affiliates Start-of-Year Balance Sheet.*

in long-term liabilities (mortgage) plus $230,250 in retained earnings and $161,050 in owners' equity. You can also see the link between the income and expense report for the same period and the year-end balance sheet. The net income on the income and expense report is shown as retained earnings on the year-end balance sheet. This is because the practice did not elect to pay any cash dividends at the end of the year and so retained net earnings as practice equity. Because the balance sheet is a picture of the practice's financial position, future transactions will change it. The retained earnings portion of the equity accounts represents owner's/shareholder's equity that is derived from retained profits at a given point in time. This equity is contributed to the practice by the shareholders/owners and represents invested capital. If owners choose to withdraw their equity, the practice's assets will decrease. To fund the withdrawal, the practice will need to obtain cash by tapping bank deposits or selling property or equipment. In a practice it is easy to see that such a withdrawal of equity would affect its ability to deliver care or maintain its technology. This is the reason that, in a young practice, attention should always be paid to the expectations of the investors for return on their invested funds. If investors are satisfied with their returns, they will allow the practice to retain invested capital until the practice can sustain equity withdrawals with no compromise in quality of care.

### 10.4. Understanding Cash Flow and Its Effect on the Balance Sheet

Our previous discussion has shown the relationship between the income and expense statement and the balance sheet. The statement of cash flow and the balance sheet are also interdependent. In fact, the statement of cash flow translates the net income, shown on the income and expense statement, into a clear picture of the practice's cash position. The indirect cash flow analysis requires two balance sheets, one at the beginning of the period and one for the end, and an income and expense statement for the beginning of the period. The cash flow analysis examines the sources and uses of cash in the business in three activity areas: operations, investing, and financing.

Figure 10.3 shows the results of comparing two balance sheets—one at the beginning of the fiscal year and one at the end. The net income reported at the start of the fiscal year was $230,250, shown in Figure 10.1.

Based on the cash flow analysis (Figure 10.3) and start-of-year balance sheet data (Figure 10.2), the balance sheet at the end of the year would look as shown in Figure 10.4.

| Cash Flow Categories | Balance Sheet Data— Beginning and End of Year Comparison | Cash Effect | Source or Use of Cash |
|---|---|---|---|
| Operations | Increase in Accounts Receivable: $50,000 | ($50,000) | Use |
| Operations | Increase in Inventory: $20,000 | ($20,000) | Use |
| Operations | Depreciation expense for period: 7% straight line on value of equipment | $14,070 | Source |
| Operations | Increase in Accounts Payable: $10,000 | $10,000 | Source |
| Operations was a net user of cash during this period. | *Cash was used to purchase inventory, and reduced cash was owed, apparently, to the increased number of days in accounts receivable. The practice depreciated its equipment by 7% but spent no cash to do this. It also lengthened the time it takes to pay its suppliers and thus kept some cash instead of paying its bills.* | ($45,930) | Net use |
| Investing | Increase in Equipment: $20,000 | ($20,000) | Use |
| Investing was a net user of cash during this period | *Cash was used to purchase equipment for $20,000* | ($20,000) | Use |
| Financing | Decrease in Mortgage Loan $20,000 | ($20,000) | Use |
| Financing | Cash Dividends to Investors $10,000 | (10,000.00) | Use |
| Financing | Cash in Certificate of Deposit: $10,000 | 10,000 | Source |
| Financing was a net user of cash during this period | *Cash was used to pay off the mortgage loan and to provide investors a cash dividend. The certificate of deposit was cashed in and was a source of $10,000 cash that offset the dividends paid to investors.* | ($20,000) | Use |

**FIGURE 10.3.** *Illustrative Cash Flow Analysis for a Fiscal Year.*

## 10.5. The Financial Position of a Practice: Financial Statements and Ratios

Based on an examination of the two balance sheets for the practice, it would appear that there are no serious concerns. The practice has increased its value by 14 percent over the last year and the retained earnings have increased. It has retired its mortgage debt and has purchased some new equipment. This seems to be a picture of a successful and well-managed practice. There are however, some worrisome trends. We can already see from the cash flow analysis (Figure 10.3) that the practice was a net user of cash during the last year. According to the cash flow analysis, the accounts receivable more than doubled while accounts payable increased by 28 percent. In fact, the only source of cash from operations was the depreciation expense, which is not a dependable source of funding. Depreciation represents the amount of money the business must save to replace equipment at the end of its useful life. The practice also used cash for investing in new equipment and for retiring its remaining mortgage debt. This may be an investment to support a more favorable cash position in future years, but there is some cause for concern in the near term. The practice has maintained a favorable equity position because the equity increase was funded by additional retained earnings and not by additional investor contributions. The fourth financial report, which outlines the change in owners' equity, provides this information to the investors in the practice.

The following chapter will introduce financial ratio analysis, a powerful tool to support in-depth understanding of the practice's financial position. Financial ratios capture the relationship between standard financial reporting categories and performance. They also help compare the performance of one business with another in the same peer group. Lenders use ratios such as debt-to-equity to evaluate a practice's ability to manage debt or to examine its financial management effectiveness.

| Assets | | Liabilities and Owners' Equity | |
|---|---|---|---|
| **Current Assets** | | **Current Liabilities** | |
| Cash | 2,100 | Accounts Payable | 45,900 |
| Petty Cash | 100 | Interest on Debt | 2,900 |
| | | Wages Payable | 8,500 |
| Accounts Receivable | 90,500 | Taxes Payable | 6,100 |
| Inventory | 51,000 | | |
| **Long-term Assets** | | | |
| Property | 180,000 | Owner's Equity | 161,050 |
| Equipment | 206,930 | Retained Earnings | 306,180 |
| **TOTAL ASSETS** | **530,630** | **TOTAL LIABILITIES + EQUITY** | **530,630** |

*FIGURE 10.4. General Practice Affiliates End-of-Year Balance Sheet.*

### 10.6. Concept Checkout

Be sure you understand these concepts before you begin the discussion questions:

- Generally accepted accounting principles
- Financial Standards Accounting Board
- International Standards Accounting Board
- Balance sheet
- Income and expense statement
- Cash flow analysis
- Statement of change in shareholders' equity
- Net revenue
- Accrual basis
- Cash basis
- Basic accounting equation
- Sources and uses of cash
- Depreciation

### 10.7. Discussion Questions

1. You have been offered a partnership in a local healthcare practice in a suburb of a large city. You decide to review the practice's financial situation after hearing rumors that they are not doing well. List the reports you will request from the practice and provide a specific rationale for requesting each.
2. The practice has a profit-sharing plan in place for partners. Which report is the most important to determine the profit that has been earned by the practice? List at least three questions you will ask after you have examined this report.
3. You have heard rumors that the practice is "cash poor." What report will you examine to evaluate its cash position, and what categories does this report analyze? For each category, describe at least one specific question you will ask regarding the practice's cash position.
4. The practice's partners also have a 20-percent share in retained earnings as part of their salary package. What are retained earnings, and how do they differ from other sources of equity? Because the practice is in a market with increasing competition, discuss the pros and cons of accepting an equity share in place of additional salary.
5. You notice that the practice seems to be in a favorable financial position, according to its balance sheet. But its sources of cash are

largely from financing activities, such as short-term loans. The cash flow analysis shows that operations is a net user of cash. List two questions that you will ask during your interview concerning the practice's cash position.

## 10.8. References

Additional reading on the basic financial reports will reinforce your understanding. The following resources are recommended for discussion in a healthcare context.

Baker, Judith, and R. W. Baker. 2014. *Health Care Finance: Basic Tools for Nonfinancial Managers,* 4th ed. Burlington, Mass.: Jones and Bartlett. 113–20.

Ward, William J. 1994. *Health Care Budgeting and Financial Management for Non-Financial Managers.* Westport, Conn.: Auburn House. 21–37.

# General Practice Affiliates and Titus Lake Hospital: A Provider Leasing Proposal

You are a partner in General Practice Affiliates LLP. Your practice is considering an offer from Titus Lake Hospital to affiliate under a provider leasing model. In this model, the practice retains ownership and management rights but agrees to provide primary care services on behalf of the hospital. The hospital bills the third-party payers for these services and collects the revenue. The third party pays fair-market value fees for the practice's primary care services. The provider leasing model is permitted under the Stark Act and provides complete autonomy to the practice. The hospital is a purchaser of services, and as such may require the practice to provide quality assurances and submit statements of services provided that meet the hospitals' accounting and reporting requirements.

The physician lease agreement model allows the practice to retain complete control of its business management as well as personnel and practice policies. The risks in the physician lease agreement model focus on the ability of the hospital to honor the lease agreement and pay in a timely way for services provided under the agreement. This means that the General Practice Affiliates partners must be sure that the hospital is a viable business partner in solid financial condition and that the hospital can ensure a sufficient volume to make the lease agreement worthwhile. One serious consideration in agreeing to the provider leasing arrangement is the requirement to adopt an electronic medical records system that is in use at Titus Lake Hospital. This means that General Practice Affiliates will have to invest at least $175,000 in the new system. Additional overhead costs of training staff and converting active patient records are estimated at an extra $100,000.

General Practice Affiliates has retained a financial consulting firm to

133

help evaluate the provider leasing agreement with Titus Lake Hospital. You are the health provider expert on the consulting firm's team and have been assigned to discuss the following questions in a brief analysis:

1. In your opinion, is Titus Lake Hospital a good financial partner for General Practice Affiliates? You will need to analyze the financial reports provided in order to determine the hospital's financial stability.

2. What is the level of financial resources required to support the transition from one electronic medical records system to another in General Practice Affiliates? You may assume that the practice's current medical records system is completely incompatible with the hospital's, so records cannot be transferred from one system to the other. You will need to consider the amount of investment required to convert to the new system and transfer at least 750 patient records.

3. Given the existing capital structure of General Practice Affiliates, what is your recommendation for financing the purchase of the new medical records system? You may assume that the practice has been able to retain some investors and service its current debt.

4. If General Practice Affiliates decides to attract investors to finance a new medical records system, what return on investment do you think would be reasonable? Consider the current economic environment as relevant to this decision.

5. Discuss the risks inherent in the provider lease agreement with Titus Lake Hospital and recommend at least three risk management strategies to the partners in General Practice Associates.

Case Exhibit 1 contains the financial statements for Titus Lake Hospital for two years and the cash flow analysis for the current year. Case Exhibit 2 has the financial statements for General Practice Affiliates.

## Case Exhibit 1

| Titus Lake Hospital (350 beds) | | | |
|---|---|---|---|
| *Balance Sheet, as of Dec. 31, 2011 and 2012 ($1,000)* | | | |
| | | | |
| | **2011** | | **2012** |
| *Assets* | | | |
| 1. Cash | 72,000 | | 70,100 |
| 2. Accounts receivable (net) | 14,000 | | 16,500 |
| 3. Prepaid expenses | 200 | | 100 |
| *4. Current assets (1+2+3)* | *86,200* | | *86,700* |
| 5. Land, buildings, and equipment, at cost | 305,000 | | 320,000 |
| 6. Accumulated depreciation | 25,000 | | 31,000 |
| *7. Land, buildings, equipment, less depreciation (5-6)* | *280,000* | | *289,000* |
| **8. TOTAL ASSETS** | **366,200** | | **375,700** |
| | | | |
| | | | |
| *Liabilities and Fund Balance* | | | |
| 9. Accounts payable | 13,100 | | 15,900 |
| 10. Short-term loan payable | 1,400 | | 1,000 |
| 11. Mortgage payable, current | 8,500 | | 8,500 |
| *12. Current liabilities (9+10+11)* | *23,000* | | *25,400* |
| 13. Mortgage payable and other debt, long-term | 213,800 | | 210,500 |
| *14. TOTAL LIABILITIES (12+13)* | *236,800* | | *235,900* |
| | | | |
| 15. Fund balance | 129,400 | | 139,800 |
| | | | |
| **16. TOTAL LIABILITIES AND FUND BALANCE (14+15)** | **366,200** | | **375,700** |
| | | | |
| | | | |
| *Income Statement, 2012 ($1,000)* | | | |
| | | | **2012** |
| *a. Patient service and other revenues* | | | *360,000* |
| | | | |
| b. Expenses | | | |
| c. Salaries and wages | | | 170,000 |
| d. Supplies | | | 67,000 |
| e. Depreciation | | | 31,000 |
| f. Interest | | | 13,000 |
| g. Other | | | 38,200 |
| *h. Total expenses (c+d+e+f+g)* | | | *319,200* |
| | | | |

| i. Excess of revenue over expenses | | | 40,800 |
|---|---|---|---|
| | | | |
| | | | |
| *Cash Flow Analysis 2012 ($1,000)* | | | |
| | | | **2012** |
| Sources of cash: | | | |
| From operations: | | | |
| Excess of revenue over expenses: | | | 40,800 |
| Adjustments to convert to cash basis: | | | |
| I. Depreciation expense | | | 31,000 |
| II. Accounts receivable change | | | 2,500 |
| III. Prepaid expenses change | | | (100) |
| IV. Accounts payable change | | | 2,800 |
| *V. Net cash generated from operations* | | | *77,000* |
| | | | |
| Uses of cash: | | | |
| VI. Payment on short-term loan | | | 400 |
| VII. Payment on current portion of mortgage | | | 0 |
| VIII. Acquisition of land, buildings, and equipment | | | 15,000 |
| *IX. Total cash used during period* | | | *15,400* |
| | | | |
| **X. Net change in cash during period** | | | **61,600** |

## Case Exhibit 2

| General Practice Affiliates Balance Sheet 2012 | | | |
|---|---|---|---|
| **Assets** | | **Liabilities and Owners' Equity** | |
| **Current Assets** | | **Current Liabilities** | |
| Cash | 2,100 | Accounts Payable | 45,900 |
| Petty Cash | 100 | Interest on Debt | 2,900 |
| | | Wages Payable | 8,500 |
| Accounts Receivable | 90,500 | Taxes Payable | 6,100 |
| Inventory | 51,000 | | |
| **Long-term Assets** | | | |
| Property | 180,000 | Owner's Equity | 161,050 |
| Equipment | 206,930 | Retained Earnings | 306,180 |
| **TOTAL ASSETS** | **530,630** | **TOTAL LIABILITIES + EQUITY** | **530,630** |

| General Practice Affiliates Income and Expenses 2012 | |
|---|---:|
| **Category** | **Amount in dollars** |
| **Operating Revenue** | |
| Direct Patient Services | 700,000 |
| Health Promotion Counseling and Classes | 200,000 |
| Prisoners Health Contract | 100,000 |
| **Total Operating Revenue** | 1,000,000 |
| **Operating Expenses** | **1,000,000** |
| **Direct costs** | |
| Salaries | 300,000 |
| Contract labor | 100,000 |
| Supplies including stock pharmaceuticals | 75,000 |
| *Sub-total—direct costs* | *475,000* |
| **Indirect costs** | |
| Mortgage Payment | 80,000 |
| Insurance | 50,000 |
| Utilities | 30,000 |
| *Sub-total—indirect costs* | *160,000* |
| **Total Costs (direct + indirect costs)** | **635,000** |
| **NET REVENUE FROM OPERATIONS** | **365,000** |
| (Total Operating Revenue minus Total Costs) | |
| **Other Income (Expenses)** | |
| Loan Interest paid | (80,000) |
| Earnings Before Taxes | 285,000 |
| Income Taxes | (42,750) |
| Business Taxes | (12,000) |
| **NET REVENUE** | **230,250** |

## General Practice Affiliates Cash Flow Analysis 2012

| Cash Flow Categories | Balance Sheet Data— Beginning and End of Year Comparison | Cash Effect | Source or Use of Cash |
|---|---|---|---|
| Operations | Increase in Accounts Receivable: $50,000 | ($50,000) | Use |
| Operations | Increase in Inventory: $20,000 | ($20,000) | Use |
| Operations | Depreciation expense for period: 7% straight line on value of equipment | $14,070 | Source |
| Operations | Increase in Accounts Payable: $10,000 | $10,000 | Source |
| Operations was a net user of cash during this period. | *Cash was used to purchase inventory, and reduced cash was owed, apparently, to the increased number of days in accounts receivable. The practice depreciated its equipment by 7% but spent no cash to do this. It also lengthened the time it takes to pay its suppliers and thus kept some cash instead of paying its bills.* | ($45,930) | Net use |
| Investing | Increase in Equipment: $20,000 | ($20,000) | Use |
| Investing was a net user of cash during this period | *Cash was used to purchase equipment for $20,000* | ($20,000) | Use |
| Financing | Decrease in Mortgage Loan $20,000 | ($20,000) | Use |
| Financing | Cash Dividends to Investors $10,000 | (10,000) | Use |
| Financing | Cash in Certificate of Deposit: $10,000 | 10,000 | Source |
| Financing was a net user of cash during this period | *Cash was used to pay off the mortgage loan and to provide investors a cash dividend. The certificate of deposit was cashed in and was a source of $10,000 cash that offset the dividends paid to investors.* | ($20,000) | Use |

# Section 6

# CHAPTER 11

# Financial Performance Evaluation

## 11.1. Chapter Objectives

After completing the chapter you should be able to:

1. Explain the use of ratio analysis in comparing an organization's financial performance to internal and external benchmarks.
2. Define liquidity, solvency, and profitability ratios and state their purposes in financial analysis of an organization.
3. Discuss the relationship between key ratios and the practice's financial performance with regard to return on assets and return on equity.

## 11.2. Financial Ratios as an Analytical and Comparative Tool

The basic financial statements we discussed in the previous chapter provide basic documentation of a practice's financial situation in three ways:

- The balance sheet reports the assets an organization controls and how they are financed at a given point in time.
- The income and expense statement reports the money the organization earned and spent over a specified time period.
- The cash flow statement (also called statement of changes in financial position, or SCFP) reports the organization's sources and uses of cash over a specified time period.

These financial statements follow a standardized format that conforms to generally accepted accounting principles defined for U.S.

businesses. Because these statements are standardized and report on a consistent set of financial parameters, they can compare a practice's performance over time (otherwise referred to as longitudinal comparisons), or they can compare one practice with another. Internal comparisons of a practice with its previous performance require less contextual adjustment than comparisons of one practice with another. For example, internal comparisons over time generally represent a relatively homogenous set of environmental and internal factors. Major changes in the practice's environment or internal management are known and can be accounted for in longitudinal comparisons. In external comparisons of the practice with others, differences in environment and management approaches may not be known and cannot be controlled for in the analysis. True peer grouping of similar practices for comparison purposes is quite difficult. This is why external comparisons should be used with some degree of caution. External financial performance benchmarks are provided for use by several organizations. The Medical Group Management Association (MGMA) provides benchmarking resources for medical practices as well as training materials at its website, www.mgma.com/benchmarking. Materials are geared to physician practices but provide general guidelines for all primary care practices. The Risk Management Association provides financial analysis services to the banking and credit industries. The group provides an annual statement benchmarking service for its members using North American Industry Classification System (NAICS) codes. NAICS codes are also used by federal agencies to classify U.S. businesses for regulatory and financial reporting purposes. The 2012 NAICS code for independent practitioners other than physicians is 62139. This code includes independent offices of various health practitioners from naturopaths to registered nurses. For nurse practitioners providing primary care, a closer comparator might be 621111, Offices of Physicians (Except Mental Health Specialists). The difficulty of matching nursing care to the appropriate NAICS codes illustrates the challenge of finding a peer group for comparing financial performance across practices.

## 11.3. Ratio Categories and Their Purposes in Financial Analysis

Table 11.1 presents four common ratio categories that are used to understand and compare the financial management of a business.

These ratios are commonly used by organizations that valuate physician practices such as credit and banking organizations. Internal management of practices may include factors such as practitioner productivity ratios that look at the relative value units (RVUs) delivered per practitioner, or the total weekly (or monthly) visits per practitioner. In

TABLE 11.1. Four Common Ratio Categories.

| Ratio Group | Purpose | Ratio | Definition |
|---|---|---|---|
| Profitability | Measures the organization's ability to generate enough net revenue to provide a return on investment and maintain and upgrade its infrastructure to continue delivering quality healthcare. | Profit margin | Net income/Total revenue |
| | | Return on assets | Net income/Total assets |
| | | Return on investment | Net income/Equity |
| Liquidity | Measures the ability of the organization to convert its non-cash assets into cash. | Current ratio | Current assets/Current liabilities |
| | | Quick ratio | Cash + marketable securities (if any) + net accounts receivable/Current liabilities |
| | | Accounts Receivable | Total accounts receivable/Gross fee-for-service charges × (1/12) (*MGMA Definition*) or Net accounts receivable/Sales revenue × 365 |
| Long term solvency ratios | Long-term (more than 1 year) financing of the practice, which indicates how it financed itself (use of debt or invested capital) and its ability to meet its loan obligations, that is, to pay interest and principal payments. | Debt/Equity | Total liabilities/Total equity |
| | | Leverage | Assets/Total equity or Debt/Total equity +1 |
| | | Long-term debt/Equity | Non-current liabilities/ Total equity |
| | | Times interest earned | Number of times earnings exceed interest payments: Earnings before interest and taxes/Required interest payments |
| Asset Management or Activity Ratios | The level of effectiveness in the practice's use of assets. | Asset turnover | Operating revenues/Total assets |
| | | Fixed-asset turnover | Operating revenue/Net fixed assets |
| | | Inventory turnover | Operating revenue/Inventory |

practices that derive revenue from procedures, the practitioner's productivity in conducting procedures may also be examined. If RVUs are not used, caution should be exercised in looking at productivity because complexity of the procedure or visit needs to be accounted for. In addition to productivity, internal managers may also be concerned with payer mix. MGMA provides one set of analytical tools for understanding reimbursements by payer mix as well as comparative external benchmarks. Payer mix is a component that may be useful in very competitive markets where the practice makes choices regarding specific contracts.

Both practitioner productivity and payer mix are secondary analytics that may provide explanations for financial outcomes that do not meet expectations or compare favorably with external benchmarks. In general, the main approach to financial evaluation should consist of the ratios presented in Table 11.1. Depending on the results of this first-level analysis, the practice may need to examine additional indicators such as productivity or payer mix. It may also decide to consult with a financial management expert.

## 11.4. Basic Ratio Relationships and Financial Performance Diagnosis

Financial ratios describe important relationships between the financial components presented in the basic financial reports. Financial ratios highlight several critical questions: (1) What financial relationship does the ratio represent? (2) What ratio values and trend indicate favorable financial performance? (3) What financial management strategies are suggested to improve the ratio? In the following example we will consider these critical questions in the context of the asset turnover ratio, an important indicator of practice activity. We will analyze each financial ratio using the questions to understand the financial relationships inherent in the ratio measurement.

*1. What financial relationship does the ratio represent?*

This ratio measures the ability of an organization to use its assets effectively and earn net income. It is computed by dividing the total revenue on the income and expense statement by the total assets the organization owns. The analyst should be careful to note that the ratio does not consider expenses or asset management. Asset turnover is focused only on the central question of how effectively the practice uses its total asset base to earn revenue. It does not examine the details of the asset base, the payer mix, or other details of revenue management. These important process components are vital contributors to the aggregate outcome of asset turnover but are not measured directly with this ratio.

## 2. *What ratio values and trend indicate favorable financial performance?*

In the case of asset management, the larger the value of the ratio, the more favorable is the financial performance. For example, if the practice has an asset management ratio of 1, this indicates that for every one dollar invested in assets by the practice, one dollar of revenue is earned. In general terms, this means that all assets are at least returning the value that was invested in them after depreciation. If the ratio moves below 1, the practice needs to question the efficiency of asset use in the practice. Depreciation of fixed assets is a consideration because a new practice with no depreciation will need to earn comparatively more revenue to have a favorable asset turnover than an older practice that has depreciated assets. The underlying consideration in this analysis is that newer assets should perform more efficiently than older ones. However, new healthcare practices may not yet have an established payer base capable of generating stable revenue. In addition, healthcare practices as small businesses must make comparatively high investments in fixed assets such as electronic medical record systems or diagnostic technology in order to begin offering services. The required high investment together with the time it takes to establish a reliable payer mix may require new practices to accept lower than average asset turnover rates at the start.

## 3. *What financial management strategies are suggested to improve the ratio?*

It is helpful to determine not only the value of the ratio but also its direction. This may require tracking the ratio over time to determine if the trend is improving. In the case of asset turnover, it is possible to track monthly, quarterly, or semiannual values to determine the trend. After the practice determines the trend and understands its magnitude and direction, managers compare it with the best available industry norms for a peer group. Then the practice can define strategies to improve the ratio. One way to begin formulating a financial strategy is to deconstruct the ratio into its components and analyze contributing elements to each one. Practices sometimes consult financial management professionals who can offer strategic financial advice. Before hiring a consultant, the practice should conduct a thorough internal analysis and discuss the findings. This usually maximizes the value of the consultant's time and ensures better results.

The technique of concept mapping can be helpful when breaking down financial ratios into their contributing factors. In the case of asset turnover, here is a simple concept map for each ratio component.

*Operating revenues* are affected by factors such as:

- Contractual service agreements
- Payer mix
- Expense management and budgeting
- Provider productivity (RVU/provider)
- Patient satisfaction
- Market competition
- External environmental factors

*Total assets* are affected by factors such as:

- Age of the asset base
- Technology intensity of the practice (required investment in technology)
- Decisions regarding ownership versus leasing of major assets, inventory management, and cash management
- Capital budgeting and acquisition management strategies

Analysis of each concept by the managers and members of the practice can provide an important basis for correcting asset management strategy. It is particularly important to understand which factors are controllable within the practice and which are not. For example, external environmental factors such as a severe economic recession can affect the total revenue of a practice but is not within the control of the practice. However, once the practice understands the external factor, internal strategies that can be controlled such as provider productivity need to be monitored and corrected as patient demand slows.

Each of the key ratios can be monitored, analyzed, and used to guide the financial strategy. It is critically important for the practice to be aware of these indicators and use them effectively to support financial survival and success.

The interaction of financial indicators is also an important analytic tool. The DuPont system of ratio analysis suggests some key interactions that are useful to the financial manager.

The key assumption underlying the DuPont analysis is that the goal of any enterprise is to maximize return on investment. Healthcare providers frequently debate this assumption in the context of healthcare delivery, which is an essential human service that needs to be available to all. However, in previous discussions we have argued that return on investment is a critical parameter for the practice's survival in the free-market environment of U.S. healthcare. The saying "no margin, no mission" expresses the dual strategy of the healthcare industry exposed to market forces. Investors will not make monetary resources available to provide healthcare services if their investment does not yield returns. Therefore, if the healthcare practice cannot assure investors an adequate return, they will withdraw their financial support and the practice may need to borrow and earn revenue to service the debt. Debt is usually more costly and certainly riskier than funding the practice using investments. The return on investment in any financial enterprise is related to financial ratios as follows:

*Profit margin × Asset turnover = Return on assets*

*Return on assets × Leverage = Return on investment*

The first ratio relationship basically states that the *return on assets* is a product of profitability multiplied by the efficiency of asset use. A practice that is able to retain a large share of its revenue may decrease its return on assets by using its asset base inefficiently. Looking at the numerical relationships demonstrates this. If the profit margin is 10 percent and the asset turnover is below 1, it is easy to see that the return on assets is decreased.

*Profit Margin (0.10) × Asset Turnover (0.5)*
*= Return on Assets of (0.05)*

In this example, the money the practice retains in net income (profit margin) is reduced by 50 percent due to the inefficient use of assets.

The second part of the DuPont computation tells us that return on assets is multiplied by the ratio of assets/total equity. For example, if the firm finances every dollar of its assets with equity, Return on Assets is multiplied by 1, that is the financing of the firm's assets does not affect the ROA. If, however, the firm introduces some debt into the financing of assets, the amount of assets in the firm increases beyond the equity in the firm. In short the firm uses borrowed money to acquire assets rather than only funds provided by the investors in the firm. If the firm earns a positive return on these assets, then investors gain an added benefit, that is money is earned by the firm using funds provided by lenders, not investors. The value of the firm increases and investors benefit by the firm's use of borrowed funds.

*Return on assets (0.05) × Leverage (1.5)*
*= Return on investment (0.084)*

In the above example, the firm has improved the return on equity by using some borrowed funds to finance assets. Caution should be introduced into the decision to improve investor's return on equity using borrowed funds. Certainly financing productive assets with funds provided by lenders would be preferred by investors, as long as the practice services the debt without increasing the risk to quality and the practice's survival. The decision to borrow funds should always be made with full consideration of the heightened risk that accompanies the increased return on equity gained. Careful examination of the cash flow analysis is a vital part of the ratio analysis because this report shows clearly the effect of debt service on the practice's cash position.

## 11.5. Concept Checkout

Be sure you understand these concepts before you begin the discussion questions:

- External financial performance benchmarks
- NAICS codes
- Profitability ratios
- Liquidity ratios
- Asset management ratios
- Long-term solvency ratios
- DuPont system of ratio analysis
- Relationship of asset turnover to net income
- Relationship of leverage to return on investment

## 11.6. Discussion Questions

1. You are considering accepting a partnership in a primary care practice. You have been provided with a set of financial reports that include the balance sheet, the income and expense statement, and the cash flow analysis. Identify at least four financial ratios you will examine to help decide if you are going to join the practice. Provide a rationale for the ratios you have selected.
2. Conduct a DuPont analysis using the financial statement presented in Chapter 10. Based on this analysis, would you recommend that the practice assume more debt? Why or why not?
3. You wish to compare the financial performance of your nurse practitioner-owned primary care practice, which is focused on health promotion. Which NAICS code will you use for this practice and why?
4. Define the concept of peer grouping for the purposes of financial

analysis. Propose at least three questions that would guide your selection of an appropriate peer group.

5. Your investors state that they require a 7 percent return on investment or they will withdraw their invested funds from your practice. You have been asked to present a case for accepting a 4 percent return for the next five years at the next board meeting. List three main points to support your case.

## 11.7. References

Additional reading on financial ratios can be found in the following resources:

Baker, Judith, and R. W. Baker. 2014. *Health Care Finance: Basic Tools for Nonfinancial Managers,* 4th ed. Burlington, Mass.: Jones and Bartlett. 121–28.

Ward, William J. 1994. *Health Care Budgeting and Financial Management for Non-Financial Managers.* Westport, Conn.: Auburn House. 31–37.

# CHAPTER 12

# Projecting Financial Performance

## 12.1. Chapter Objectives

After completing the chapter you should be able to:

1. State the purpose of the pro forma financial analysis in management of an organization or project.
2. Use financial evidence to define the pro forma objectives.
3. Describe feasible financial actions that can be taken to achieve defined objectives.
4. Discuss barriers and supports for achieving defined financial objectives.
5. Describe financial interrelationships and their impact on strategy.

## 12.2. The Pro Forma Financial Analysis: Purpose and Use

Our discussions to this point have focused on understanding the past financial performance of the practice. Financial statements and ratios are based on past performance and help owners understand how their practice has done financially. After they understand past performance, the next step is to project future financial performance. Owners can use the same analytical tools—key financial ratios and relationships— for future projections. This type of analysis is typically done in two cases:

1. At the end of a financial reporting period when the accounts for the period are closed and the financial reports become available. At this point the practice can project future financial performance and analyze the impact of these projections on critical financial ratios.

Necessary operational and financing actions can be planned based on the pro forma analysis.

2. When the practice is facing a major change in the external environment or in capital structure, such as a large business loan or investment. In this case the practice is well advised to examine a set of pro forma financial statements that incorporate the proposed changes, either in the environment or in the capital structure, to see if other changes should be made to ensure financial sustainability. Frequently, several forces act together to motivate the practice to make major changes. For example, regulatory changes from the Affordable Care Act have made capital investments in electronic medical records necessary for most practices. A practice facing such a major investment decision must also consider the potential regulatory impacts on its financial outcomes. For example, in order to qualify for phase-two meaningful use bonus payments from the U.S. Department of Health and Human Services, the practice must electronically exchange information with at least two government agencies. So the practice must consider the cost of this exchange or risk losing the expected bonus payments. In either case, the pro forma analysis is an important step in understanding the future situation for the practice.

In summary, the purpose of the pro forma analysis is to understand financial outcomes based on future conditions. The analysis informs strategic planning and problem solving. It is typically conducted at the end of a fiscal year or ahead of major environmental and financial changes.

### 12.3. Using Evidence to Build the Pro Forma Analysis

A practice earns revenue by providing services. In previous chapters we discussed reimbursement analysis and revenue planning. They form the essential starting point for pro forma analysis. Revenue is interrelated with income, expenses, assets, and liabilities. As revenues increase, the practice may see a rise in accounts payable as it needs more supplies, pharmaceuticals, and staff. Proforma analysis first looks at the factors that affect revenue of healthcare practices. Table 12.1 presents some of these factors and the evidence that defines accurate revenue projections.

After the practice has examined factors likely to impact future billing and income, the pro forma revenue can be projected. This will inform the estimates of the net revenue and the most revenue-sensitive items on the balance sheet: accounts receivable, inventory, accounts payable, and retained earnings.

TABLE 12.1. Factors Affecting Practice Revenue.

| Revenue Factor | Evidence |
|---|---|
| Healthcare reimbursement policies for major payers in the practice environment. | Medicare payment policies as proposed in the semiannual Medicare Payment Advisory Commission (MedPac) reports to Congress. |
| | Medicare payment policies as enacted by Congress and subsequent regulations as published by the Department of Health and Human Services. |
| | State Medicaid reimbursement policies as defined by legislatures and state Medicaid agencies. |
| | Private-sector health insurance reimbursement policies as defined by major payers in the practice environment. |
| | Federal and state regulations concerning the uninsured, medically indigent, and self-paying consumers of healthcare. |
| Demand for healthcare services in the practice market area. | Population data on demographic, economic, and education information for the practice's market area. |
| | Data on the major employers in the practice's market area, including those that self-insure or do not provide health insurance to employees or certain employee categories. |
| | Seasonal employment trends and labor migration factors for the practice's market area. |
| | Major shifts in employment in the practice's market area, for example major business openings and closures. |
| | Data on the health of the population in the market area, including the prevalence of chronic disease and injuries, immunization coverage, and stability of the population. |
| Health sector workforce | Average wages for the major categories of healthcare workforce likely to be needed by the practice. |
| | Labor trends and supply of healthcare workers employed or projected to be employed by the practice. |
| Technology | Technology needed by the practice based on demand and labor analysis. Trends in technology already used by the practice but likely to require significant upgrades or changes. Regulatory trends likely to impact practice technology such as electronic medical records, new confidentiality or records management policies, or other administrative changes impacting information technology or information transfer. |

## 12.4. Building the Pro Forma Financial Plan

The pro forma estimates of accounts receivable can be based on historic levels of receivables adjusted for new payers or new payment policies by established payers. For example, if the practice has conducted a careful reimbursement and revenue analysis and estimates that monthly billings will be $500,000, then the historic trend in the accounts receivable ratio can be examined and applied to estimate the receivable billing for a defined period of time. This estimate will need to be adjusted based on the revenue factors discussed in the previous section. For example, if a major public payer such as Medicaid passes a new policy that extends the allowable time to pay providers from 45 to 60 days, the historic receivables trend will need to be adjusted before the pro forma receivables estimate is done. In healthcare markets with adverse employment trends such as business closings or layoffs, it is reasonable to assume that time to collect self-payment accounts, required deductible payments, and co-payments will increase. Bad debt losses can also reasonably be expected to increase, and this will be reflected in accounts receivables and projected retained earnings.

Retained earnings are also affected by the practice's dividend policy. The expectations of investors regarding return on investment will be affected by prevailing interest trends in the capital markets as well as in the average dividends that an investor could earn on an investment of similar risk in the stock market. Healthcare practices need to examine their dividend policy at the time they build their annual pro forma estimates and update the policy based on industry and broader economic trends. Neglecting this review can result in unexpected requests for withdrawal of funds by investors, which can destabilize the practice. Once the dividend policy has been defined for the upcoming year, the net income can be adjusted by the amount to be allocated for dividend payments. The retained earnings reported on the pro forma balance sheet reflect the portion of net income not paid to investors.

Inventory and accounts payable are interrelated items that are sensitive to practice revenue because they reflect the volume-sensitive requirements for supplies, stock pharmaceuticals, and non-capital technology purchases. Historic estimates of the value of inventory reported on the balance sheet should be adjusted for current demand and technology estimates in order to arrive at the pro forma inventory estimate. Anticipated major changes in demand as well as adjustments in the cost of non-capital technology purchases (e.g., minor equipment) should adjust the historic estimate of inventory. Accounts payable generally depend on the value of inventory, and this pro forma estimate can be obtained by looking at the historic behavior of payables against inventory. As with inventory estimates, major changes in the supplier's payment policies are an adjustment factor for the estimate based on historic trends.

Table 12.2 shows the pro forma balance sheet with revenue-sensitive items highlighted. In order to complete the pro forma balance sheet, the practice needs to estimate its future cash position. As with other estimates, the cash position can be estimated based on historic trends either by looking at the average cash position over the last five years or by looking at the trends in a ratio such as cash/net revenue, or the percent of revenue held in cash. Changes in management policy within the practice also affect the cash position estimate. For example, some practice managers like to hold a more liquid position to compensate for unexpected labor costs in an unstable labor market. If the practice forecasts an increase in the need for contract or other short-term labor, it may adjust its cash position estimates to allow for more liquidity in the future and reflect this in the pro forma estimates.

The pro forma balance sheet can now be finalized. Changes in long-term assets and long-term liabilities are completely within the practice's control and can be determined from the strategic plan. Any strategic plan to acquire additional capital assets and the planned financing for them should be reflected in this part of the pro forma balance sheet. Projected taxes and debt service will derive from defined government and lender policy, and any changes in these policies should be considered. The final projected pro forma balance sheet is the future projection of the financial situation of the practice in the coming fiscal year. As we have learned in previous chapters, the statement of changes in financial position (sometimes called the sources and uses of cash) can also be derived from the pro forma balance sheet that has been built.

TABLE 12.2. One-Month Budget for Ambulatory Care Practice.

| Assets | | Liabilities and Owners Equity | |
|---|---|---|---|
| Current Assets | | Current Liabilities | |
| Cash | 2,100 | Accounts Payable | 35,900 |
| Petty Cash | 100 | Interest on Debt | 2,900 |
| Certificate of Deposit | 10,000 | Wages Payable | 8,500 |
| Accounts Receivable | 40,500 | Taxes Payable | 6,100 |
| Inventory | 31,000 | Long-term Liabilities and Equity | |
| Long-term Assets | | Mortgage | 20,000 |
| Property | 180,000 | Owners' Equity | 161,050 |
| Equipment | 201,000 | Retained Earnings | 230,250 |
| Total Assets | 464,700 | Total Liabilities + Equity | 464,700 |

## 12.5. Financial Barriers and Supports: SWOT Analysis

Once the pro forma balance sheet is complete, the practice needs to conduct a critical examination of the assumptions made in the context of internal strengths and weaknesses (SW) and external opportunities and threats (OT). The strategic advantage of adding the SWOT analysis to the pro-forma process is considerable because the assumptions used to build the pro forma are largely based on historical data supported by known environmental factors. In a dynamic healthcare environment the practice's ability to respond to a rapidly changing environment greatly impacts its financial performance. The SWOT analysis enhances this ability.

The Practice's internal strengths and weaknesses can be assessed using a facilitated group discussion that focuses on a careful analysis of past performance. Many practices do not have the time or resources for this discussion format, and in this case a consensus-building approach known as the Delphi method can be used. According to this method each member is asked to list the practice's strengths and weaknesses responding to a series of questions that guide the assessment. One excellent approach to structuring a participant response is to ask each member of the practice to identify strengths and weaknesses in the areas of access to care, cost of care, quality of care, and, optionally, patient satisfaction. Once the responses are received, the top-rated five to seven answers in each category are compiled. Then in a second survey, participants rate the top-rated three items in each category for strengths and for weaknesses. In the final round, the three highest-scoring strengths and weaknesses are listed for each category, and the practice members are asked to rate the top strength and the top weakness. Data from the three rounds of the Delphi survey are then used to construct a matrix that presents each item according to the level of consensus about its contribution to the practice's strengths and weaknesses. The most widely shared (consensus-based) strengths and weaknesses form a relevant context for the pro forma projections: the practice can focus on the strengths to support and weaknesses to remedy to best achieve the proforma targets.

The environmental opportunities and threats can be derived from the research conducted to adjust the historical estimates for the pro forma projection. Table 12.1 provides a good framework to support definition of the environmental opportunities and threats relevant to the pro forma projections. The practice needs to make a strategic decision concerning the management of its environment. Some practices make no attempt to impact its environment; others devote considerable resources to external activities that influence the environment. Examples of activities that shape the environment include membership in professional and civic organizations, and on professional and regulatory boards, formal and informal lobbying of state and federal elected officials, and service in regulatory and policy oversight organizations specific to healthcare delivery. If a SWOT analysis is carefully conducted, the practice can shape its environmental outreach to impact the most important opportunities and threats in its immediate environment. For example, if the SWOT analysis highlights a major layoff by a key local employer, the practice can work with state and local officials to ensure some continuation of health benefits for unemployed workers. This type of effort preserves some practice revenue while ensuring primary healthcare services for newly unemployed workers.

The resources and time required to conduct a SWOT analysis in conjunction with pro forma projections represent a critical investment in good future financial performance as well as a contribution to the social welfare of the practice's community.

## 12.6. Financial Interrelationships and Financial Strategy

As with the past-performance ratio analysis discussed in Chapter 11, the financial interrelationships represented by the DuPont analytical system are useful for adjusting strategy after estimating pro forma financials. The first part of the DuPont system defines the relationship between two major financial ratios:

$$profit\ margin \times asset\ turnover = return\ on\ assets$$

Profit margin is defined as the ratio of net income to total revenue. The component parts of net income are shown on the income and expense statement as total revenue minus total costs. Total revenue is composed of revenue from operations plus revenue from nonoperating sources. Expenses include all operating expenses shown on the income and expense statement. Thus:

$$(operating\ income + nonoperating\ income) - operating\ expenses = profit\ margin$$

Asset turnover is defined as operating income/assets. The component parts of asset turnover are fixed assets such as property and equipment added to current assets such as inventory, accounts receivable, and cash. This suggests that the DuPont relationship can be represented in a four-part relationship composed of (1) total revenue, (2) total assets, (3) net revenue, and (4) equity. These are the components required to yield the critical return on equity to the investor. Here is the proof of this four component relationship for the return on equity:

$$total\ revenue/total\ assets \times net\ income/total\ revenue$$
$$= net\ income/total\ assets = ROA\ [Return\ on\ Assets]$$

$$ROA \times total\ assets/equity\ [\text{termed Leverage}]$$
$$= net\ income/equity = ROI\ [Return\ on\ Investment]$$

The practice can analyze the pro-forma projections using the DuPont system to determine if the critical components of total revenue generation, expense control, asset efficiency, and strategic use of debt to multiply the investor's resources are all present. The financial interrelationships between these critical components are defined by the DuPont formula. As discussed in the previous chapter, inefficient use of the assets can result in an asset turnover below 1, which effectively reduces the return on investment because net profit margin is multiplied by asset turnover to give the ROA. If revenue is maximized and expenses are under control resulting in a favorable net profit margin but the practice has invested in too many assets that do not produce revenue, then the ROA is reduced. If the asset base produces revenue equal to or exceeding the value of the assets, then the ROA is increased by the efficiency with which the practice uses assets. This interrelationship is a critical point for most practices to examine.

The second interrelationship is the use of some debt to leverage the investment of the practice owners. In very risk-averse practices, debt is not used and all assets are financed with investor's money. This means that there is no multiplier to increase the return on investment. If the practice adds some debt to its asset financing and it continues to use assets efficiently and control expenses, then the return on investment is increased or multiplied because the relationship of total assets to investment. After the pro forma financials are created, analysis of the critical interrelationships is a useful step in either assuring continued good performance or correcting financial problems that are impacting service to clients.

## 12.7. Concept Checkout

Be sure you understand these concepts before you begin the discussion questions:

- Purpose of the pro forma financial analysis
- Critical factors that affect the pro forma analysis
- Revenue-sensitive components of the pro forma balance sheet
- SWOT analysis applied to pro forma projections
- Delphi method

- Contribution of expense control, asset efficiency, and leverage to return on investment
- Return on investment

## 12.8. Discussion Questions

1. You have been asked to give an in-service to all practice professionals about the need for pro forma analysis. List at least three critical points you want to make during this in-service and the explanations you will use to support these points.
2. The practice is interviewing financial consultants to assist them in building pro formas required by the bank before a loan for an electronic medical records system can be approved. Suggest two critical questions to ask during the interview and give rationales for asking these particular questions.
3. The consultant has delivered the pro formas to the practice. Describe at least one additional analysis that you will suggest using the pro formas, and outline the steps you suggest to accomplish this analysis.
4. The practice investors have requested a meeting with the practice owners to discuss the financial strategy of the practice for the next year. You have been asked to discuss the return on investment strategy of the practice based on the pro forma data provided by the consultant. Outline the method you will use to present the projected return on investment.
5. A practice owner has suggested that the practice borrows the money to purchase the electronic medical records system proposed for the next year. The practice currently uses no debt, so its asset/equity ratio = 1. Discuss at least three potential effects on financial performance resulting from the decision to use debt.

## 12.9. References

The best resources on pro forma financial statements in the context of strategic planning can be found at the website of the U.S. Small Business Administration. The document called "How To Write a Business Plan" contains many valuable suggestions about strategic planning for an existing business. The document is available at www.sba.gov/sites/default/files/How%20to%20Write%20a%20Business%20Plan.pdf.

# Provider Financial Goals and Management

You have learned that financial ratios can provide useful indicators to the financial management and outcomes of a healthcare practice. They can also be used in conjunction with pro forma financial reports to design goals to be met in the future.

In this case you are going to design a financial plan for General Practice Affiliates LLP based on the assumption that they have accepted the provider leasing agreement that you analyzed in Case 5. The focus in this case analysis is on the current and future financial ratios that you will recommend as indicators to be monitored as the provider leasing agreement moves forward.

Please review the situation and exhibits in Case 5, and then answer the following questions regarding present and future (pro forma) financial ratios.

1. What major ratio categories will you select for financial indicators to monitor as the provider leasing agreement moves forward? Suggest at least three ratio categories, state your rationales for these suggestions, and describe the direction you expect ratios in these categories to move if the leasing agreement is successful.

2. Analyze General Practice's current situation using the key ratios you have suggested.

3. Provide evidence from the literature on the amount of change you expect to see in the ratio categories you have selected. Discuss the variables that might be expected to impact these ratios given the physician leasing agreement and the adoption of the new electronic medical records system.

4. Suggest at least one ratio per category and a pro forma target ratio to achieve in the future. For example, if one of your ratio categories is liquidity, you might suggest a target current ratio (current assets/current liabilities) of 1.2.

5. For each of the three pro forma ratios you have suggested, list measures that will be needed to reach your recommended proforma targets. Support your recommendations with evidence from the healthcare finance and practice literature.

# Section 7

# CHAPTER 13

# Project Financial Management: Planning and Budgeting

## 13.1. Chapter Objectives

After you complete this chapter you should be able to:

1. Describe the steps necessary to develop financial plans and budgets for projects.
2. Discuss one example of an integrated project management strategy.
3. Develop an integrated project management plan and define the project team.
4. Define a project financial plan using financial performance indicators.

## 13.2. Project Financial Planning and Budgeting

The previous chapters in this book have discussed the financial issues involved in establishing and managing an ambulatory care practice. The basic financial infrastructure, budget, evaluative financial reports, and financial planning tools have been introduced. The next two chapters will focus on financial planning for capital investment projects in an established practice.

Unlike ongoing funding for the organization's professional and business routine, a project targets a special set of objectives, operates on a set-aside budget, keeps separate track of activities and costs, and involves project-specific reporting and evaluation requirements. If the practice will have to invest significant capital in order to implement the project, the first financial consideration should be the feasibility of the capital investment. In highly regulated industries such as healthcare, the decision to invest capital in a major project may be mandated (and incentivized) by a regulatory or corporate partner rather than the provider's discretion. For example both Medicare and Medicaid have incentive programs to encourage adoption of electronic medical records (EMRs). Starting in 2015, Medicare providers that are eligible to but do not adopt EMRs will pay a penalty. There is no such penalty for Medicaid providers, but there is an incentive program to encourage adoption of EMRs (see www.cms.gov/Regulations-and-Guidance/Legislation/ EHRIncentivePrograms/Downloads/Medicaid-EHR-Guide.pdf). At the time the program began, EMRs were not common in small to medium ambulatory care practices. The transition required significant funding and expertise that was frequently not part of the practice's core staff. Whether a practice continued with manual files or transitioned to EMR, the core business of patient care carried on. This example illustrates a capital investment decision encouraged by a regulator. Other investments may be suggested by practice partners, staff, or patients.

Regardless of the proposed project's origin, the decision to implement it has financial, management, and quality implications. Two critical questions distinguish a capital investment project from ongoing business: (1) Is the proposed investment large when compared to the annual budget of the practice? (2) Will a significant period of time (usually more than one year) elapse until the beginning of returns on the investment?

Not all investments should be considered capital projects. Investments that require significant additional capital, time, and management before realizing any returns  deserve careful consideration as capital investment projects.

The financial data inputs to the capital investment decision require the application of some of the tools and strategies that you have learned in previous parts of this book. For example, the first task in capital investment planning is to clearly define the project so it can be financially evaluated. The best way to accomplish this is to require a project proposal with a structured definition and a detailed analysis of costs and benefits to the practice. Project proposals are expensive and time-consuming. Frontloading a small- or medium-sized practice with the requirement to develop a complete project proposal may be a waste of time if the project is not adopted. Burdened with preparation a full-fledged proposal, practice staff would decide to forgo additional projects thus leaving valuable improvement initiatives unrealized.

An alternative course of action would be to write a brief concept paper that outlines one or several projects and use it to highlight potentially viable ideas that merit further consideration. External funding agencies frequently request concept papers prior to proceeding with full proposals. The main components of a concept paper are: (1) a statement of the project's purpose or goal; (2) a brief summary of the project, including its objectives, major implementation stages, and expected measurable outcomes; (3) an overview of costs that specifies the major cost items; and (4) an overview of organizational supports required to implement the project.

The major financial concern at the start of designing the project is cost, and the costing strategies you studied in Chapter 6 will be useful here. Most project costs can be estimated by predicting the direct costs and then adding an overhead percentage that recognizes the indirect costs. Project overhead typically includes items such as physical plant, utilities, administrative support, including financial management, and maintenance services. Establishing the percentage for indirect costs can be complex and lengthy. For example, the U.S. Department of Labor specifies several methods for establishing the Negotiated Indirect Cost Rate Agreement (NICRA) for organizations applying for federal grants and contracts (see http://www.dol.gov/oasam/programs/boc/costdeter-minationguide/cdg.pdf). These methods require careful examination of the practice's financial statements to determine which costs are indirect and which are direct. A portion of the organization's total overhead costs are approved for allocation to a federally supported grant or contract if that overhead is involved in any project. A practice may use a similar but less detailed process to arrive at a percentage of indirect cost to allocate to a proposed internal project. Table 13.1 illustrates two methods of indirect cost allocation to a project budget.

*Method 1:* Indirect expenses can be apportioned to a project according to a reasonable allocation method as presented in column C and explained in column D. This is the accurate approach. However, in most cases the overheads are not easily traceable to a project, particularly at the planning stage. For example, an administrative assistant's time and the practice's floor space would often be used for a multitude of ongoing and project-specific activities alike. Telephone and electricity bills can be analyzed for project-specific phone calls and energy consumption, however, at an effort that is hardly worth a marginal gain in accuracy. Hence,

*Method 2:* An organization-wide pool of indirect expenses (column B) is estimated from the income and expense statement. The total of direct and indirect expenses (line 12) is divided by direct expenses (line 11) to produce the loading factor, which shows the excess of total costs over direct costs for the practice as a whole. This loading factor would be uniformly applied in project-specific budget estimations. For each new project the direct costs will be estimated as accurately as possible;

TABLE 13.1.  *Estimating a Project's Indirect Costs.*

| A. Expense Category | B. Organization | C. Project Expense | D. Reasonable Allocation Strategy and Other Comments |
|---|---|---|---|
| 1. Direct costs | | | |
| 2. Salaries | $300,000 | $75,000 | Project as % of total salaries (25% of organization salary base) |
| 3. Contract labor | $100,000 | 0 | 0 |
| 4. Indirect (overhead) costs | | | |
| 5. Administrative salaries | $100,000 | $25,000 | Project as % of total salaries (25% of organization salary base) |
| 6. Mortgage payment | $80,000 (6,000 sq. feet) | $13,333 (1,000 sq. feet) | Project as % of total square footage (1,000 / 6,000 = 1/6; 1/6 × $80,000 = $13,333.33) |
| 7. Property insurance | $50,000 | $8,333 | Project as % of total square footage (1/6 × $50,000 = $8,333.33) |
| 8. Utilities | $30,000 | $5,000 | Project as % of total square footage (1/6 × $30,000 = $5,000) |
| 9. Building maintenance, including janitorial services | $10,000 | $1,667 | Project as % of total square footage (1/6 × $10,000 = $1,666.66) |
| 10. Indirect cost subtotal | $270,000 | $53,333 | Sum of lines 5 to 9 |
| 11. Direct cost subtotal | $400,000 | $75,000 | Sum of lines 2 and 3 |
| 12. Total costs (direct + indirect) | $570,000 | $128,333 | Line 10 + Line 11 |
| 13. Loading factor: ratio of total costs to direct costs | 1.68 | 1.71 | Line 12 : Line 11 |

then the total direct costs will be multiplied by the loading factor to yield the estimated total costs of a given project.

Whether organization should prefer to use method 1 or method 2 depends on a variety of circumstances: (1) A breakdown of total costs into direct and indirect costs: If the practice accounts for most of its costs as direct costs, the remaining (indirect) costs can be spread across the ongoing and project activities by using the same loading factor. This uniform allocation approach will not cause a major discrepancy between the actual and financed costs. However, if indirect costs account for a significant share of practice costs, their allocation to a project should be as accurate as possible, just because of their sizeable volume. (2) If the project is financed externally, the funding party may balk at an apparently high loading factor, arguing that project-specific funding must not be diverted to finance the practice's overhead. To make the cost proposal defensible, the practice should have a meticulous proof of the estimated loading factor. Method 2 would be instrumental in this case. (3) Project sponsors do not like the overhead rate to appear above the average in a peer group. They would be right to raise questions if the same applicant comes up with significantly different loading factors in their project proposals or grant applications over a relatively short period of time. Regardless of the method, a practice should be sensitive to a client's concerns and flexible enough to adjust its estimates to the client's requirements. Of overriding importance is the value-for-money principle of project financing: the share of indirect costs should be at a competitively low rate; the higher the rate, the higher the funder's expectations of the value of the project deliverables, and the practice should be prepared to meet those expectations. At the same time, the practice cannot afford to lose money due to underestimated costs. A possible reconciliation between cost realism and competitive project budgets may lie in a carefully planned cross-subsidization of projects and core activities in an established practice. Cross-subsidization, if critically needed, requires a judicious approach: it must not result in a financial strain on the practice's core business, which would affect volume and erode the quality of healthcare.

To summarize, the methods of indirect (overhead) cost assessment in the project budget recognize that projects will require some general resources from the practice in the major categories of space, utilities, and administrative staff and that there are real costs associated with these resource needs. The cost detail required is simple enough to allow project proposals to be developed with a small costing effort while still assuring that the major overhead expenses are accounted for. Guidance is provided to any member of the staff assembling a project concept paper or proposal that 68 percent of the total direct costs of the project should be added to compensate the practice for the overhead required (line 13, column B, Table 13.1). Once the total direct costs of the project are computed, 68 percent is added to the final budget number to compensate the practice for indirect costs. This is the project budget that will be approved for concept consideration and proposal purposes. There are frequently negotiations about the required percentage of indirect costs because project staff is always seeking a competitive advantage with external funders. The practice needs to be clear that adding more staff and space has a cost effect that must be recognized and reimbursed. After the initial concept paper is reviewed and approved, the project proposal is developed. This is the basis for a "go" or "no go" decision. Once the funding organization has accepted the project, the detailed application for external support is usually completed. This may be a federal or state grant application or an application for investment or debt financing. In many cases there is a combination of both sources of capital to fund projects. Careful costing and adequate overhead calculations are important to ensure that the project is sufficiently capitalized for successful implementation. Under-capitalization of projects results in a shortfall of resources vis-à-vis project objectives and is a common reason for project failure.

## 13.3. Accounting for Project Expenses

The suggested strategy to integrate project financial management into the practice is to establish a modified fund accounting structure to support project fiscal accountability without including the project into the core accounts of the practice. Projects are expected to have sufficient revenue from donors, grants, investments, or loans to meet direct and indirect expenses, but they are not expected to produce a return on the investment during the implementation phase. Blending the project into the main chart of accounts would create a distorted view of the practice revenue and expense, which would likely decrease the return on investment estimate for the main business of providing care. Establishing a separate fund and financial reports for the project ensures that if the project does not meet its expenses, the practice will be aware of this immediately and an explicit decision can be made to either subsidize the project or discontinue it. Use of this "stove-pipe" (project-by-project) fund accounting approach makes project financial management clear and eliminates the risk of unwarranted spillover of costs to the core business of the practice.

Project fund accounting requires that the practice assign the project a fund name and number and that all project costs are traceable to that fund. The agreed-on indirect cost allocation is applied to the direct project cost at regular intervals, either monthly or quarterly. It appears as a cost category on the project's expense statement. Fund accounting also produces separate budget and variance reports and a clear analysis of the project's performance against its budget.

Reports from the project manager to the practice owners should occur at regular intervals, and any unfavorable budget variances should be discussed and remedied as quickly as possible. Explicit subsidization of the project due to budget overruns need to be considered in a fiscally responsible way, and a strategic management decision made to continue or discontinue the project. This decision is typically made based on the importance of the project and its overall goals, objectives, and benefit to the practice as a whole.

## 13.4. Integrated Project Management Plan and Team

Integrating the project financial management into the practice using the fund approach means that the project becomes a business within the larger practice. The project has its own set of deliverables that meet the defined goals and objectives. For the project to meet its goals and objectives, the practice needs to define a project management plan and a team that is clearly responsible for project performance. Small projects may have part-time staff and may share staff with the practice. This is a fact of life for small- to medium-sized practices that want to implement projects. However, care should be taken that project staff build a team identity and understand that they are responsible for the project's success. Projects that are not adequately staffed and lack identity become orphans that no one owns and for which no one is accountable. These projects usually fail to deliver results and frequently become a financial drain. But two important steps help keep tabs on project costs.

1. Staff accountability for project time is the key device in a toolkit of financially disciplined project management. The implementation plan should provide a detailed list of relevant activities. Project staff should charge their time to specific activities, entering hours by date and activity charge codes in weekly or bi-weekly timesheets. Staff whose workload is split between practice and project activities should record their time accordingly. Separate charge codes for the main practice cost centers and for the project should be issued. Project staff should be trained to report hours actually spent on each activity so that practice management has a clear idea of the time expended on project implementation. Labor variances can then be accurately reported on the monthly budget reports and action taken quickly if actual project labor varies unfavorably from budgeted labor.
2. Financial accountability with the focus on the project budget should be established and reinforced with periodic reports of budget allocations and variances. Project funds should not be blended with the core business funds and should be accounted for using the project-specific fund accounting approach.

The practice's project team needs support and assistance to understand new reporting requirements such as timesheets and expense tracking. This is typically a point of resistance for practices that have not previously required timesheet reporting or expense tracking. The project staff frequently sees the additional accountability requirements as a tax on their time. Careful management preparation and support builds the project team and invests them with a clear sense of accountability for the project and its results. An effective way to accomplish this is to allow the team to report project progress and challenges to the practice management on a regular basis. All members of the project team should be present during these reports and contribute actively to the discussion. The project's financial impact on a practice can be beneficial if the project team is clearly accountable for results within the established project cost structure.

## 13.5. Project Financial Management

Approval of a project and receipt of funding initiates the financial management cycle. At this point the practice assigns a fund number to the project and defines a chart of accounts that recognizes any requirements that the funding source has for project expenditures. In the project fund, the indirect cost can be applied as an aggregate charge once it is approved by the funder and the practice. The practice owners, project managers, and financial team need to decide if project cash will be pooled or kept in a separate bank account. For small projects, managing a separate account may not be justified. Table 13.2 presents the advantages and disadvantages of each approach to managing project cash.

The practice needs to incorporate by reference any expense control policies that are a condition of project funding. For example, many projects that are funded by external sources restrict travel costs or modes of travel. These terms and conditions need to be incorporated into the project financial policies so staff is aware of and compliant with them. Project financial staff should introduce any audit safeguards that prevent overspending in areas constrained by external spending policies because funders view cost overruns as a serious issue. The U.S. General Accounting Office publishes the Federal Acquisition Regulations, which illustrate some of the common safeguards and the requirements that concern external funders (see www.gpo.gov/fdsys/pkg/CFR-2002-title48-vol4/pdf/CFR-2002-title48-vol4-chap3.pdf).

The fund account may be classified as a special use fund, a capital investment fund, or a private purpose fund. Consult with the accounting service or bookkeeping staff to designate the appropriate classification. The fund must be in compliance with any external requirements set

TABLE 13.2. *Managing Project Cash: Pooled Versus Separate Approaches.*

| Pooled Cash Management—One Bank Account for Both Practice and Project | Separate Cash Management—Separate Bank Accounts for Practice and Project |
|---|---|
| Reduces the need to account for cash transfers from one account to another. | Ensures that project and practice funds are clearly separate. |
| Lowers banking costs because one main account is used for all banking transactions. | Facilitates separate authorizations for spending because signature authorities can differ for each account. |
| Decreases the risk of insufficient funds in the project account due to delayed payment from the external funder. | Provides a clear audit trail from bank cash accounts to internal project fund accounts. |
| Reduces accounting reconciliations to banking accounts. | Ensures a careful review before project and practice funds are transferred because separate transactions are required. |
| Transfers between practice and project funds can be handled through interfund transfers rather than a cash withdrawal and deposit into separate banking accounts. | |

by the funding source. Once the fund is established, a number of management policies and principles should be defined to ensure competent fund management.

1. *Authorization.* Individuals authorized to spend from the fund may differ from those authorized for the general practice. Ensure that fund authorizations are consistent with project responsibilities.
2. *Control.* Set control levels for the fund that are consistent with the external funder's requirements and the conditions of the grant or project funding. For example, if the purchase of major equipment is prohibited as a condition of funding, then the account controls should be consistent with this policy.
3. *Segregate incompatible duties.* An incompatible duty allows one individual to create an irregular transaction and then conceal it with another transaction. For example, no one individual should have the authority to authorize a payment, process a check, sign a check, and reconcile the bank statement with the internal accounts.
4. *Review.* The review of the fund should be done in the context of the project deliverables, goals, and objectives. Because the fund is defined to serve a specific purpose, review of the fund should be completed in the context of the specified deliverables. The review frequency should be sufficient to ensure that the project is progressing as defined in the proposal.

5. *Budget variance.* Conduct the budget variance review in the context of the project goals and objectives rather than with reference to organizational goals. For the purposes of budget variance review, the project is a stand-alone financial entity with no resources beyond its funding. The critical question in budget variance review should be focused on completion of deliverables within the defined cost parameters.

## 13.6. Concept Checkout

Be sure you understand these concepts before you begin the discussion questions:

- Capital investment project
- Capital investment planning
- Project proposal
- Project concept paper
- Indirect cost allocation
- NICRA
- Fund accounting
- Pooled cash management
- Fund management policies

## 13.7. Discussion Questions

1. The state health department has issued a call for proposals to design and implement a diabetes education plan for adolescent women on Medicaid. The diabetes educator who is a part-time consultant to your practice has requested support to write the proposal. The three-year project is funded at $750,000. Your net revenues last year were $850,000 on an account base of $2 million. Your practice management team is meeting to consider the request. Draft a recommendation outlining a process for deciding whether to support this project.

2. Congratulations! Your practice was awarded the diabetes education project and the educator has been designated as the principal investigator. Outline three critical questions that you would like to see answered in a presentation to the practice management board.

3. You are meeting with the practice financial management team to design the project's financial framework. What financial management approach will you recommend and why?

4. Identify one major risk-management strategy that you will recommend to the financial management team.

5. The diabetes educator has requested the involvement of the consulting endocrinologist to provide personalized care planning for adolescent women who cannot control their blood glucose levels. The project does not have funds to pay for personal medical care. How do you recommend that this request be handled?

## 13.8. Reference

The classic discussion of project evaluation and management may be found in:

Brealey, Richard A., and Stewart C. Myers. 2003. *Brealey & Myers on Corporate Finance: Capital Investment and Valuation.* New York: McGraw-Hill. 223–55.

# CHAPTER 14

# Project Financing and Valuation

## 14.1. Chapter Objectives

After you complete this chapter you should be able to:

1. Define project financial flows based on the integrated project plan.
2. Compare and contrast the main methods of project valuation.
3. Define the steps in the net present value analysis of projects.
4. Discuss the impact of the discount rate in project evaluation.
5. Evaluate project decisions based on project valuation analysis.

## 14.2. Constructing Project Financial Flows

Projects can be developed based on the practice's needs for a new service or technology, or the practice can respond to a request from an external funding agency for a defined deliverable. The previous chapter introduced a flexible definition of a project and the considerations that are important to presenting it. In this chapter we will focus on understanding the financial flows and valuation of projects.

The term *cost-benefit* is frequently heard in healthcare. The method to financially valuate a project is essentially a practice-focused cost-benefit analysis. There may well be benefits that accrue to the community, but such benefits are not considered in this analysis. Neither are the costs that might have to be accepted by the community if the practice undertakes certain types of projects. For example, a common phenomenon encountered by growing practices is community impact of practice development. As the practice grows it requires community infrastructure support such as overflow parking, pedestrian safety, neighborhood lighting, and security. These considerations might not have been needed when the practice was small. If the practice offers additional services like drug rehabilitation or mental health treatment the community may notice a different type of client visiting the practice and using adjacent community resources. All of these changes confer real costs on the community, and an expanded cost-benefit analysis that considers all stakeholders may be requested. The method for conducting this analysis is the same as the method we will learn for a practice-focused project cost-benefit analysis. The difference is in the amount of data that must be collected and considered in the analysis. For purposes of learning the relevant financial techniques, we will limit our discussion to costs and benefits traceable to the practice itself.

The previous chapter discusses the general approach to project financial management using fund accounting. In this method the indirect expenses that the project must pay to the practice to support practice-wide overheads are allocated as a percentage of the project direct costs or total budget. The same approach will be used for the financial projections that need to be developed for project financial flows.[1] Table 14.1 illustrates this method and includes an allocated overhead expense determined by the method discussed in Chapter 13. The project financial flows are illustrated on a five-year diabetes education project that will be billable to the payers in the practice under both private and public insurance plans providing the conditions defined for such training are met. In particular, the Medicare program will reimburse diabetes outpatient training within certain parameters, as will most state Medicaid programs and private payers. Estimate of demand for the training is important as the starting point for predicting future revenue from the project. To estimate demand, the baseline and future practice client base (i.e., eligible population within the practice market area) should be assessed.

Table 14.1 is the product of extensive market research and costing undertaken by the practice financial and operations management staff. The cost of this research is reflected as part of the year 0 investment required in the project. The projected growth in years 4 and 5 is the result of anticipated development of contracts with the school district to provide diabetes self-management training to newly diagnosed diabetic adolescents in 15 schools in the market area. Preparation of the financial cost and financial benefit table can be very detailed and include best-

---

[1]Project financial flows are the income and expenses incurred by the project for a given period. This period may be annual or quarterly, depending on the length of the project.

*TABLE 14.1. Estimating Financial Flows by Project Year.*

| Year | # of patients | Revenue Years 1–5 | Investment Year 0 | Project Costs | Allocated Indirect Costs (23% of project direct costs) | Taxes (15% of net revenue) |
|---|---|---|---|---|---|---|
| 0 | 0 | 0 | 184,500 | 0 | 3,500 | 0 |
| 1 | 50 | 15,000 | 0 | 50,000 | 11,500 | 0 |
| 2 | 75 | 22,500 | 0 | 50,000 | 11,500 | 0 |
| 3 | 100 | 30,000 | 0 | 60,000 | 13,800 | 0 |
| 4 | 250 | 75,000 | 0 | 75,000 | 17,250 | 0 |
| 5 | 500 | 150,000 | 0 | 75,000 | 17,250 | 8,662.50 |

case and worst-case scenarios weighted by the probability that each will occur. In cases when a great deal of financial risk is involved due to the required investment, a more detailed analysis is advisable and may be required by lenders or investors. The basic procedure is exactly the same as that presented in Table 14.1. The required investment in the project is estimated and so is the projected revenues based on market and payer research. The project direct and allocated indirect costs are estimated using the costing principles discussed in Chapter 6. Finally, the project's tax burden is assessed. Notably, Table 14.1 shows that in year 5 the net revenue exceeds the cost for the first time. It is easy to see by looking at the cost projections that economies of scale are important and that management needs to direct its attention to the efficiency level projected in the cost analysis.

## 14.3. Project Valuation Methods

Table 14.2 presents the four project valuation methods commonly in use. Two of these methods take the time value of money into account, and we will consider these in greater detail. The payback and accounting rate of return are sometimes used because they are easy to calculate; but the decisions made by these methods may be incorrect depending on the underlying inflation rate in the economy. The availability of computing software that performs net present value and internal rate of return calculations suggests that these methods should always be preferred project valuation approaches. Either method ensures that the practice fully evaluates the project financial value in the context of the economic environment.This chapter will provide a detailed example of developing a net present value analysis. Many financial analysts will use the internal rate of return to value projects because it is an easily

*TABLE 14.2. Project Valuation Methods Compared.*

| Valuation Method | Valuation Basis | Practice Risk | Time Value of Money | Profitability |
|---|---|---|---|---|
| Payback | Project cash flow | Considered | Not considered | Not considered |
| Accounting rate of return | Profitability | Considered in the context of profit earned | Not considered | Considered |
| Net present value | Project cash flow | Considered | Considered | Considered |
| Internal rate of return | Project cash flow | Considered | Considered | Considered |

developed measure with a clear benchmark. The internal rate of return (IRR) calculates the project rate of discount that makes the net present value of the project equal 0. Given the cash flows projected in Table 14.1, it is not difficult to see that the project will have a negative net present value and IRR. The problem with the cash flow picture shown in 14.1 is that the project requires significant upfront investment of practice resources and does not develop sufficient volume for a positive return until year 5. Using the NPV and IRR functions available in any of the common spreadsheet programs, the calculation shows a negative net present value to the practice at a 3 percent rate of interest and no positive internal rate of return that would result in an NPV $\geq$ 0.

The value of either of these methods is that they show management clearly the decisions it must make about the proposed project. For example, the practice may feel that the project has value but that the design needs adjustment to make it financially feasible—that is, with a positive net present value and an IRR of zero at an acceptable rate of interest. Alternatively the practice can reject the project because of too

*TABLE 14.3. Project Cash Flows, $.*

| Year | Revenue | Cost | Return |
|---|---|---|---|
| 0 | 0 | (184,500) | 184,500) |
| 1 | 15,000 | (61,500) | (46,500) |
| 2 | 22,500 | (61,500) | (39,000) |
| 3 | 30,000 | (73,800) | (43,800) |
| 4 | 75,000 | (92,250) | (17,250) |
| 5 | 150,000 | (100,913) | 49,088 |
| NPV = ($279,474) | | | |

much financial risk, or it can decide to cross-subsidize the project by operating the project at a loss and compensating with earned profits in other sectors of the practice. The extent to which this is possible depends on the practice's total financial position.

Redesign of the proposed project to produce a positive net present value must focus on adjusting the revenue, cost, or timeline as well as an evaluation of the discount rate used to compute the net present value. The amount of inflation expected during the life of the project is a critical parameter to consider in net present value analysis. Lower inflation rates increase the value of a project and the time it can afford to begin to generate revenue. Higher inflation rates require revenue generation to occur sooner since inflation erodes the value of future dollars. To understand this, consider that one dollar today is worth thirty-nine cents in ten years at a 10 percent rate of inflation, while at a 1 percent inflation rate, the same dollar is worth ninety-one cents. You can easily see that the choice of a discount rate to use when valuing a project with cash flows over a period of years is critical. In the current project, it is expected that lower inflation rates will increase its value because it takes time to begin to generate returns. A graphic picture of the proposed project revenue and spending patterns illustrates this clearly and also suggests areas on which to focus to improve project valuation.

The project's cost and revenue patterns suggest that a longer valuation horizon might result in a more favorable net present value if the project can sustain the efficiencies seen in year 5. Additionally, the wide

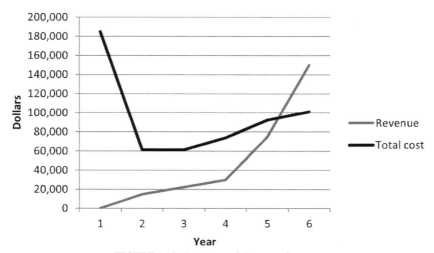

*FIGURE 14.1.* Revenue and Expense of Project.

*TABLE 14.4. NPV of Project Investment under Alternatively Defined Project Parameters.*

| Discount Rate | Net NPV |
|:---:|:---:|
| 1% | $46,849.40 |
| 3% | $24,678.33 |
| 5% | $5,689.00 |
| 7% | ($10,620.49) |
| 10% | ($30,947.00) |

difference between the total cost and revenue lines in the project's early years suggests that either the start-up costs need to be reduced or the revenue generation needs to improve earlier. The practice must decide if it can wait longer for the project to be profitable, reduce start-up costs, and achieve positive revenue flow.

Adding three years to the project, reducing start-up costs by 45 percent, and accelerating revenue flow gives the result shown in Table 14.4. The added volume of the school-based diabetes education contract, the accelerated revenue earning, and the reduced start-up costs result in a positive new present value for the project at discount rates of up to 5 percent. The planning result is that project implementation is dependent on more rapidly increasing project volume while keeping expenses and start-up costs lower and producing revenue on a more aggressive timeline. It is also important to assume that inflation will be controlled; any rate above 5 percent results in a negative value for this project. The project's pattern of cost and revenue is typical for patient education or other high start-up-cost projects in which minimum staff are needed whether class size is two or twenty.

Understanding the revenue and expense pattern in proposed projects is important not only for practice management but also for project managers and staff. It clarifies the relation of cost, revenue, and volume that is necessary for a financially successful project.

### 14.4. Impact of the Financial Environment on Projects

The financial environment surrounding a project has two components: the practice's internal financial environment and the region's external economic and financial conditions. All projects are affected by the financial situation of the practice. Financial instability will jeopardize the project, particularly in the start-up period when the new endeavor depends on the practice's support while it gains market share and begins to generate revenue. If the practice is encountering financial difficulties, the project may not be able to gather sufficient volume or retain staff long enough to become profitable. A realistic analysis of the practice financial outlook is essential to project planning once the start-up parameters and costs are clearly understood.

Another consideration for planning is the extent to which the project complements the core business of the practice. For example, the diabetes education project discussed here can be seen as a complement to the practice. It does not replace the core work of primary care practitioners, but it adds a valuable complementary service. This is particularly true if the practice has quality indicators as part of its third-party reimbursement contracts that focus on emergency admissions or readmissions for diabetics or other measures that indicate a lack of good management of diabetic conditions. By creating a more educated consumer base for the practice, the diabetes education project complements the practice and adds value. This complementarity should be an important consideration in the decision to implement a project, particularly in a small to medium practice that has little financial surplus.

The external practice's financial environment surrounding the practice is also an important consideration. In the diabetes education project, it is clear that, to become profitable, the project depends on the volume generated by the school contract. If the economic outlook for the region in which the practice is located is good, the project can reasonably expect school enrollment to be stable or expanding. If, however, the financial prospects for the region are less positive, the project might be in jeopardy because it depends on a stable or growing population of school-age children for its projected volume. Regional economic outlooks are available from a variety of sources that should be consulted when making the decision to invest in a project. This is also true when considering grant-funded projects. For example, a project that is funded by a municipal or county government should be examined carefully to be sure its returns are sufficiently stable to justify the start-up investment. In the case of state and federal projects, the stability of funding may be better, but a careful analysis of the pattern of funding and defunding similar projects and the conditions of funding continuation should be clearly understood. For example, if a federally funded project requires the practice to generate a certain level of service for funding continuation, a risk analysis needs to be done to determine how difficult it will be to generate the required volume benchmark. Considerations of demand for the project service and population stability are important variables in this analysis.

The impact of the external financial environment on a proposed project is a major planning consideration. Investing management time and resources in a clear understanding of these factors reduces the financial risk of a project and may make the difference between financial success and failure.

## 14.5. Project Financial Evaluation

The three phases of financial evaluation parallel the project life cycle: project planning, project implementation, and project outcomes. We have discussed the financial evaluation that should occur as part of the planning phase. The important aspects to consider in this start-up financial evaluation are the quality of the data on which projections are based and the evidence of the financial environments surrounding the project. After project start-up, the implementation, or process evaluation phase of the project begins. Fund accounting is the recommended way to manage financial reporting. Monthly reports of performance against budget together with variances should be provided to project and practice managers. As previously recommended, it is important that the project has an administrative home within the practice and a practice manager assigned to work with the project team. Review of the monthly fund report reflecting project finances is a good opportunity for the practice manager assigned to the project to understand the progress that is being made and discuss any unexpected problems that may arise. Besides the routine monthly financial reporting, it is useful to identify benchmarks and ask for periodic reports against these defined benchmarks. In the diabetes education project, patient volume expansion in years 3–5 is critical to success. Patient volume benchmarks can be determined on a quarterly basis and project staff can report against these volume benchmarks. Where ambitious volume expansion or complex technical deliverables are expected, it is useful to break down the expected aggregate result into a series of intermediate milestones to be monitored and reported against. This allows for corrections to be made before the project falls too far behind a critical deliverable. Enlisting additional technical or marketing support to remedy problems early can be the difference between success and failure over the defined life of the project.

Monitoring processes that are indicative of the external environment are important if the project depends on increasing participation from the community. The unexpected closure of a major employer is an example of an environmental shock that will not be overlooked if good environmental scanning is in place. Depending on the project focus, it may be advisable for senior project staff to establish certain regular external environmental monitoring activities. In the diabetes education project, senior project staff may wish to attend school board meetings to understand the strategic issues in the education sector. If the practice has an ongoing environmental assessment team, the project staff and the team should discuss monitoring activities. Important organizations such as the local chamber of commerce, municipal, county, and state governments all have public communication or outreach offices that provide regular information to interested businesses. Regular attendance at meetings and regular scanning of information about key environmental agencies should be expected of project and practice senior staff as part of the evaluation portfolio.

The practice may also want to examine the project's opportunity cost, that is, costs associated with implementing the specific project rather than doing something else. For example, resources devoted to diabetes education could as easily be devoted to smoking cessation programs or home safety education. At critical points in the project it is useful to analyze alternatives and assess the opportunity cost of using project resources in one specific way rather than another. The project's complementarity with the practice is a critical concern in opportunity cost assessment. The better the project fits with the practice, the stronger it is as a resource allocation option, compared to possible alternatives. If a project becomes less complementary to the practice, implementation should be reassessed because the cost-benefit ratio may be too high to justify.

Conclusions from the evaluation of the project's financial outcome depend on the proposed-to-actual net present value to the practice and also on projections of the project's financial sustainability. During the outcome evaluation, the project's effectiveness may also be considered. Effectiveness evaluation allows the practice to consider not only the project's financial benefit but also its impact on non-financials such as health-adjusted life years for project beneficiaries. The benefit of including an effectiveness measure in project financial evaluation is that impact can be better aligned with the community impact goals that the practice may have defined. For example, the practice may have set a strategic goal related to improving population health in its market area. The project's impact on health-adjusted life years or on reduction of disability are both important effectiveness measures that contribute to this overall goal. Effectiveness measures are also good metrics with which to judge the complementarity of the project with the practice; contribution to the practice's strategic goals and objectives is an excellent criterion to judge complementarity. Other effectiveness measures such as community goodwill, practice professional visibility, and enhanced quality are important outcome considerations. The final project evaluation should include a focused financial report that provides an analysis of performance-to-benchmarks summary and a wider environmental impact report that focuses on effectiveness measures useful for the practice as a whole.

## 14.6. Concept Checkout

Be sure you understand these concepts before you begin the discussion questions:

- Cost-benefit analysis
- Project valuation methods
- Discount rate
- Net present value analysis
- Internal rate of return
- Internal financial environment
- External financial environment

## 14.7. Discussion Questions

1. Your practice is considering a project focused on improving healthcare services for the homeless. You presently serve insured middle-class clients who work at the local university, and you contract with a managed-care plan for clients who work in a unionized light industrial plant in the area. Assess the complementarity of the proposed project with your current practice.

2. The project analysis shows that project start-up costs will be relatively high at $120,000 because additional staff will need to be hired to provide care in a nearby public housing project. Revenue generation will be slow because these clients will have to be qualified for Medicare, Medicaid or veteran's benefits. The cash flow analysis in the project is as follows:

| Current Year Start-up | Year 1 | Year 2 | Year 3 | Year 4 |
|---|---|---|---|---|
| 120,000 | (30,000) | (20,000) | 15,000 | 25,000 |

Assuming a background inflation rate of 3 percent, estimate the net present value of the proposed project and recommend either accepting or rejecting the project based on your analysis.

3. The community where your practice is located strongly supports the homeless clinic, and your environmental analysis shows that both the university and a for-profit company would be willing to contribute cash and in-kind donations. Make three financial recom-

mendations that would change your decision about project implementation, and illustrate the impact of your recommendations on the net present value calculation.

4. Outline the project financial evaluation strategy for the project implementation phase based on your revised net present value analysis and factoring in the expected in-kind and financial support of community employers. Recommend at least two financial factors you will suggest for periodic monitoring, explain your choice, and suggest financial indicators to monitor those factors.

5. It is clear that the external environmental factors are critical to the project's success. Discuss at least three environmental factors that you will monitor on a regular basis, and provide both a rationale and indicators that you recommend be incorporated in the evaluation plan.

## 14.8. Reference

The classic discussion of project evaluation and management may be found in:

Brealey, Richard A., and Stewart C. Myers. 2003. *Brealey & Myers on Corporate Finance: Capital Investment and Valuation.* New York: McGraw-Hill. 223–55.

# General Practice Affiliates Electronic Medical Records Project

You are familiar with the intent of General Practice Affiliates LLP to enter into a provider leasing arrangement with Titus Lake Hospital in the near future. As part of this agreement, General Practice must invest in a new medical records system that is compatible with Titus Lake. The practice partners at General Practice have asked you to manage this project and present them with a concept paper that will support creation of supplier bid documents and the definition of bid selection criteria. (Please refer to Chapter 13 and 14 for the information you will need to understand the project management strategy and analytics.)

Your concept paper will need the following components: (1) a statement of project purpose or goal; (2) a brief summary of the project, including its objectives, major implementation stages, and expected measurable outcomes; (3) an overview of project costs that specifies major cost drivers but does not yet present a detailed budget; and (4) an overview of organizational supports required to implement the project.

In order to design the concept paper, you will need to consult information regarding the selection and implementation of electronic medical records systems in ambulatory health care practices. You may assume that General Practice is a medium-sized primary care practice and that its current financial condition is accurately reflected in the financials presented in Case 5. In addition to the concept paper you will need to outline the steps necessary to conduct a cost-benefit analysis of the electronic medical records project. As you consider these steps remember to include the benefits that will accrue to General Practice with the addition of clients from the provider leasing agreement with Titus Lake Hospital.

A key resource for this case is:

Bates, D. W., M. Ebell, E. Gotlieb, J. Zapp, and H. C. Mullins. 2003. "A Proposal for Electronic Medical Records in U.S. Primary Care." *Journal of the Medical Information Association* 10:1. doi: 10.1197/jamia.M1097.

# CHAPTER 15

# Concluding Thoughts on the Healthcare Financial Enterprise

## 15.1. Chapter Objectives

After you complete this chapter you should be able to:

1. Discuss the relationship between finance and population health.
2. Identify the emerging trends that will affect healthcare financing.
3. Define the role of macro- and micro-financing in responding to emerging trends in healthcare.

## 15.2. The Relationship Between Finance and Population Health

Population health, one of the goals of the multibillion-dollar healthcare industry, had not been precisely defined in the United States until 2003, when Kindig and Stoddart (2003) suggested the following definition in an article in the *American Journal of Public Health*: "the health outcomes of a group of individuals including the distribution of such outcomes within the group."

The concept of population health has long been discussed in the healthcare industry. Healthcare providers strongly believed that their core business was population health and that providing healthcare services was essential to achieving that goal. Victor Fuchs, a prominent U.S. health economist whose work is discussed in this book, has clearly shown that healthcare makes only a small contribution to the health of the population (Fuchs, 1986). Healthcare providers, on the other hand, cannot imagine how the health of the population could be sustained without their services. The answer to the sometimes perplexing dilemma of population-wide versus personal healthcare lies in the area of system optimization. In the United States, we are far from optimizing our society to engender health. The challenges we face in education, environmental pollution, poverty, substance abuse, and quality of life all impact health. Until we are able to address these issues, the health of the population will inevitably be far less than optimal, and healthcare providers will need to intervene to remedy the damage. Because of upstream deficiencies in our society the need for healthcare services is real and urgent. The important resource allocation issue is whether to continue addressing healthcare needs "downstream," by providing disease-driven health services, or to shift attention to "upstream" determinants of health. If healthcare delivery consumes more and more resources to address illness caused by increasing poverty, poor education, or environmental pollution, this spending is not remedying the underlying societal problems. This paradox is becoming more pressing as healthcare spending continues to consume an ever-increasing share of the gross domestic product of the United States.

The role of macro- and micro-healthcare finance in addressing this paradox is clear. Healthcare providers need to be as efficient and effective as possible to use the least amount of societal resources to deliver personal healthcare services. This book endeavors to provide some guidance to ambulatory care providers, to enable them to use financial resources wisely and to measure outcomes as resources are expended on ambulatory care delivery. One of the recurrent themes of the book is that those who have the technical knowledge to deliver healthcare services need to understand enough about finance at the macro- and micro-level to engage in decisions about the use of resources in their practices and in the wider professional policy sphere. This is a pressing issue because resource allocation strategies to address population health must fund a broader portfolio of activities than healthcare alone. Put simply, if population health is our goal, then resources currently used in healthcare delivery are needed elsewhere. Provider's technical knowledge about population health and its intersection with healthcare needs to be fully engaged when healthcare resource allocation decisions are made either at the system level or at the practice level.

## 15.3. The Emerging Trends Affecting Healthcare Financing

There are many trends that affect healthcare financing either directly through competition for scarce funding or indirectly by increasing the need for healthcare services. The discussion that follows highlights three of these trends and their impact on healthcare financing. These are by no means the only trends that deserve our attention, but they do highlight the need for healthcare providers to look beyond healthcare delivery to understand the impact of resource utilization and financing for healthcare.

## 15.4. Aging Societies and Longevity

Figure 15.1 conveys a very sobering picture if we assume that labor and retirement policies seen in the developed world and increasingly adopted in the developing world do not change. Retirement plans were never expected to support individuals and families for almost half of their adult life, yet if an individual retires at age 65 and lives to 104, he or she might be retired for almost as long as his or her working life. This is especially true since the need for education has lengthened the time young adults need to train before they are qualified to enter the labor force as professionals. Labor economists and policy professionals are facing the perplexing problem of how to fund such lengthy retirements, particularly if illness and disability occur early in the retirement span. The challenge to population health and healthcare professionals is clear and urgent. The burden of chronic disease we see today in the elderly has to be alleviated to provide for lower severity and resource use. Our

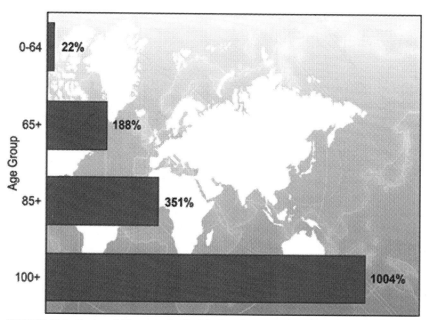

**FIGURE 15.1.** *Projected Change in the World's Population, by Age Group: 2010–2050. Source: United Nations, World Population Prospects: The 2010 Revision. http://esa.un.org/unpd/wpp.*

current concept of old age as the synonym of infirmity has to change to the concept of a healthy and productive old age. Ideally, chronic diseases that incapacitate the elderly should develop much later and be treated in ways that allow elderly individuals maximum functioning so that they remain in the workforce longer. Any other option is not financially sustainable given the demographic trends developing worldwide.

## 15.5. Worldwide Health Protection

Disease outbreaks and disasters do not respect national boundaries. The impact of these events may be devastating to nations that are impacted directly while the aftereffects would spread through the global community. For example, regional conflicts between nation-states used to be confined to the nations involved and their near neighbors. Today the refugee populations created during a regional conflict affect global population migration patterns and result in significant social cost worldwide. The effects of these refugee populations on global labor markets, national social-benefit programs, and educational systems are far reaching and economically significant.

The outbreaks of dangerous communicable diseases such as the 2003 SARS epidemic have also had profound and far-reaching impacts on people and economies around the world. These effects were presented in an important 2004 review of the epidemic published by the Institute of Medicine. The review described how effects of the epidemic centered in Asia spread throughout the world and affected the gross domestic product in most major countries both immediately and for as long as ten years (Institute of Medicine, 2004). The authors concluded that there is reasonable evidence to support rapid international intervention to control disease outbreaks in any country because the economic impacts are felt by all.

Global terrorism and its effects are familiar to everyone. In the United States, the estimated cost of the global war on terror is $758 billion through 2008 (Cordesman, 2007). While the United States may have faced the largest share of these costs, there is no doubt that the global community shares both the costs and the effects of this devastating and ongoing war. As with all conflicts, the effects of the war on terror will extend far into the future because the opportunity cost of this conflict is particularly high. The very societies that desperately need additional social spending to improve education, economic opportunity, and welfare support must divert funds to deal with terrorist groups. This distraction of funds ensures that the social conditions that engender unrest and support of terrorists will not be properly addressed.

The impact of disease outbreaks, disasters, and wars increases the likelihood that the resources needed to respond effectively to protect global health are not available. One of the few options available is to increase the efficiency and effectiveness of existing healthcare services so that resources can be redirected to prevent the disease and improve the welfare of the population.

## 15.6. The Consumer

The role of the consumer in protecting health and interacting with the healthcare system is in the midst of profound and lasting change. One of the most important of these changes is in the way consumers access and use health information. It is the rare provider who has not seen patients present Internet information that they have compiled about a health concern or care regimen. Some consumers are well informed, some use questionable information unwisely, and some do not use information at all. All of these consumers need to be assisted to a level of health literacy that will benefit them and improve their health status. Unfortunately, little of this assistance is reimbursed by health insurers.

Developing consumer health literacy is critically dependent on basic education, which has suffered from decreased funding as a result of the recession. A 2013 report by the Center on Budget and Policy Priorities shows that at least thirty-four states are providing less funding per pupil than they did before the recession (Leachman and Mai, 2013). Health and education are the main competitors for state funds, and healthcare providers are caught in the middle. As basic educational skills decline, consumers' ability to use information to improve health status is threatened and healthcare spending increases. Effective use of healthcare services depends on a reasonable level of health literacy, which depends on basic education. This circular interdependence cannot be solved without some shift of resources from healthcare to education at the state level.

## 15.7. The Roles of Macro- and Micro-Financing in Responding to These Trends

The social determinants of health include the global, national, and local environments, education, economic well-being, and social support. All of these factors interact to help consumers and households maintain health. Deficiencies in managing the social determinants raise the risk of poor health and increase the use of healthcare services. This increases healthcare costs and decreases resources available to remedy deficits in other social systems. By now this paradox is familiar to you. The solution partially depends, as we have seen, on providing healthcare effectively and efficiently, using excellent clinical skills in a quality organization that maximizes outcomes and minimizes the resources needed to achieve them.

Understanding the financial system that shapes healthcare delivery depends on knowledge of financial policy as well as organizational financial skill. This book is intended to create a base for continued learning about healthcare finance. Providers with financial skills are needed to support changes that can lead to a healthier society and a better future, not only for patients but also for those who need social services that support optimal health status at the present time, so they will need fewer health services in the future. The goal for our society is increased health and decreased healthcare.

### 15.8. Discussion Questions

1. You have been asked to make a presentation to the local chamber of commerce on population health. Outline three major points you will make about population health. For each point discuss its actual or potential impact on healthcare finance either at the system or organizational level.
2. Identify one additional development that affects healthcare financing in the United States that you would include in the list of trends. Provide evidence to support the health-financing effect and the likely impact of the trend.
3. Your healthcare practice is located in a county that intends to eliminate all after-school sports and music programs for middle school students, due to lack of funding. Outline the points that you will make in a presentation to the county board of supervisors in reaction to this proposal. Be sure to emphasize the anticipated effects on the health of middle school children and support these anticipated effects with evidence.
4. The rate of premature births to teenage mothers in your state has doubled in the last ten years. Identify one initiative that you would support to decrease this troubling trend and support your proposal with evidence of its impact. Your proposal does not need to be healthcare focused, but it does need to have direct impact on the rate of premature births to teenage mothers. You may address either the numerator (premature births) or the denominator (teenage pregnancies) in your answer.
5. You have been asked to serve on an advisory group to improve population health in your state. The group's first project will be to investigate the determinants of health for people and prioritize five

initiatives most likely to improve health. Select any state you wish and propose a prioritized list with evidence supporting each initiative you recommend.

## 15.9. References

Cordesman, Anthony H. 2007. "The Uncertain Cost of the Global War on Terror." Center for Strategic and International Studies. http://csis.org/files/media/csis/pubs/080907_thecostsofwar.pdf.

Fuchs, Victor R. 1986. *The Health Economy.* Cambridge, Mass.: Harvard University Press.

Institute of Medicine. 2004. "Learning from SARS: Preparing for the Next Disease Outbreak." Workshop Summary. http://www.iom.edu/Reports/2004/Learning-from-SARS-Preparing-for-the-Next-Disease-Outbreak-Workshop-Summary.aspx

Kindig, David and Greg Stoddard. 2003. "What Is Population Health?" *American Journal of Public Health* 93: 380–83.

Knobler, Stacey, Adel Mahmoud, Stanley Lemon, Alison Mack, Laura Sivitz, and Katherine Oberholtzer, editors. 2004. *Learning from SARS: Preparing for the Next Disease Outbreak, Workshop Summary.* Washington, D.C.: National Academies Press.

Leachman, Michael and Chris Mai. 2013. "Most States Funding Schools Less Than Before the Recession." Center on Budget and Policy Priorities. www.cbpp.org/files/9-12-13sfp.pdf.

# Index